PARADISE

Dr. Dave Hnida

GENERAL

RIDING THE SURGE AT A COMBAT HOSPITAL IN IRAQ

SIMON & SCHUSTER PAPERBACKS
NEW YORK   LONDON   TORONTO   SYDNEY

Simon & Schuster Paperbacks
A Division of Simon & Schuster, Inc.
1230 Avenue of the Americas
New York, NY 10020

First Simon & Schuster trade paperback edition May 2011

SIMON & SCHUSTER and colophon are registered
trademarks of Simon & Schuster, Inc.

For information about special discounts for bulk purchases,
please contact Simon & Schuster Special Sales at
1-866-506-1949 or business@simonandschuster.com.

The Simon & Schuster Speakers Bureau can bring authors
to your live event. For more information or to book an event,
contact the Simon & Schuster Speakers Bureau at
1-866-248-3049 or visit our website at www.simonspeakers.com.

Designed by Davina Mock-Maniscalco

Manufactured in the United States of America

10 9 8 7 6 5 4 3

The Library of Congress has cataloged the hardcover edition as follows:
Hnida, Dave.
Paradise General : riding the surge at a combat hospital in Iraq / Dave Hnida.
    p. cm.
1. Iraq War, 2003-—Hospitals. 2. Iraq War, 2003-—Medical care. 3. Hnida,
Dave. 4. Surgeons—United States—Biography. 5. Iraq War, 2003-—Personal
narratives, American. 6. Military hospitals—Iraq—History—21st century.
8. Counterinsurgency—Iraq—History—21st century. 9. Iraq War, 2003-—
Participation, American. I. Title.
        DS79.764.U6H58   2010
        956.7044'37—dc 22
    [B]   2010004056

ISBN 978-1-4165-9957-9
ISBN 978-1-4165-9958-6 (pbk)
ISBN 978-1-4391-0040-0 (ebook)

To Mothers and Fathers

CONTENTS

PARADISE GENERAL

I'M NOT A SOLDIER
BUT I PLAYED ONE IN IRAQ

THE LAST TIME I talked with my dad was on a sweltering April evening in 2004. It was a lopsided conversation. He had died of a heart attack almost thirty years earlier. But he was one of the main reasons I was hiding in a sandy ditch in the middle of Iraq, and I had some things to tell him before I died. My dad was a good man, although up until a few days before his death, I didn't always think so. A hard-toiling factory worker, he drank a fifth of cheap whiskey every day, was a mean drunk, and always left me searching for the answer to why any man felt the need to retreat to the safety of the bottle. I had my hints and theories, but never walked in his shoes, or in this case, his Army boots. It took three hours in a ditch to get a first-hand revelation about why the liquor cabinet was permanently open while I was growing up.

As a twenty-three-year-old infantry lieutenant at Anzio in World War II, my dad sent a number of other young men into battle and could never forgive himself for the ones who didn't return. This member of the "Greatest Generation" was silent about his war until

1

he abruptly and permanently corked the bottle in late 1975, when I was a senior in college.

We were driving from Newark to Philadelphia down the Jersey Turnpike when he threw a couple of quarters into a tollbooth, saying, "That's not much of a toll in this life, Dave."

I wasn't sure what he meant until a painful flood of war memories suddenly spilled from a place deep in his soul. He had never told anyone, including my mom, about any of his wartime experiences. I was the typical college kid who thought I could handle anything the world dared throw at me, but was humbled into silence as each mile marker brought a new and horrible description of the savagery of war.

In a calm and measured voice, my dad told me about being hit with flying body parts as German artillery shredded the men next to him in a foxhole; driving a knife into the throat of a wide-eyed enemy soldier no older than himself; then sending out on patrol a man, no, a boy, really, who had saved his life in an ambush only the night before. A boy whose machine-gun-riddled body my dad dragged back to American lines a few hours later. Finally came the worst story of all: the fear. The fear of failure. The fear of letting your fellow soldiers down. The paralyzing fear of fear itself. Fear was my father's lifelong bartender.

The drive ended in exhausted silence an hour later when he dropped me in front my apartment at the University of Pennsylvania. His voice was steady for the entire trip but as the car braked to a stop, his eyes were damp. With the exception of drunken bursts of anger, it was the most emotion I had seen from my father in my twenty-one years. We shook hands, said our goodbyes, and that was it. Almost. As he rolled up his window, my dad quietly said, "I'm sorry, Dave. I hope I wasn't a bad father." He died of a heart attack four days later.

I think my dad died a more peaceful man, but for me, his stories of war delivered anything but peace. I tried to make sense of the things he had told me in the hour-long monologue, wondering how his experiences shaped him and—as a result—me. And I simply couldn't shake the last words I would ever hear from him, a questioning statement that was almost a plea for forgiveness. *How could I think of him as a terrible father after what he'd been through?* I saved myself from a lifetime of regret when I answered with a smile and a quick thumbs-up as he pulled away from the curb.

As the decades following that car ride melted away, the stories did not—they seemed to be on a constant simmer below the surface of my life. I went on to medical school, got married, and started a family. Yet as I watched my own four children grow, there was always a sober thought that the only way to learn what made my father tick was to leave them, and go to war myself.

Now, in a classic case of *be careful of what you wish for,* I found myself lying in some nameless ditch along the side of a nameless road outside a village whose name I couldn't pronounce. It was a beautiful desert night, with a sparkling sky and a moon so brilliant it made me the perfect silhouette.

"Doc!" The voice came from behind in a stern whisper.

"Get your ass down and make yourself small!"

A wiry young sergeant had silently wiggled up beside me.

"You're going to get us all killed unless you get the fuck down and eat some sand, sir."

He was right. Here I was, a forty-eight-year-old doctor, well schooled in medicine but clueless in the ways of war. And fortunate to be getting lessons from a twenty-three-year-old tutor carrying an oversized M4 automatic rifle. *Christ, this kid is the same age as my father when he crawled around Italy in 1943.*

My night in the ditch had actually started hours before the sun went down. We were on our way back from convoying a wounded Iraqi insurgent from our aid station to a British combat hospital. I was nearing the end of my deployment and had been through a few close calls. Now I needed my luck to hold out for just one more ride. I stared out the small window of our Humvee as we weaved and dodged well-hidden IEDs, trying to make sense of why we were risking our skins to save the life of an insurgent who had cursed and spit on us as we loaded his stretcher into the ambulance.

Along the route, our convoy picked up a number of stragglers, vehicles whose drivers knew there was safety in numbers. Among the group of wheeled hitchhikers were a number of fuel trucks, appetite-whetting targets for anyone with a rocket-propelled grenade. The convoy hauled ass toward our base, making good time until one of our Humvees unexpectedly let out a series of groans and weakly chugged to a halt in the middle of the road. The breakdown left us no choice but to sit and wait for help. And wait we did, watching the sun disappear, and darkness creep up.

It didn't take long for word to make its way to the wrong ears that an American convoy was stranded on an isolated road. At first we could vaguely see, then only hear, scrunching footsteps in the darkening fields and groves that ran along both sides of the road. The contractors from the fuel trucks huddled as the soldiers set up a protective perimeter around the dead convoy. I settled into my spot in a ditch that was two feet deep, cradling an M16 rifle, and waited. And listened as the scrunching slowly and steadily got louder. *I'm a doctor. What the hell am I doing here? And what will my kids do when they get the news I was killed?*

As MY FOUR children grew, I made sure their world was different from the one where I grew up. They would never never worry about their father stumbling around drunk in public or throwing an empty booze bottle at their heads. And they'd never cower in a corner waiting for the alcohol to trigger an artificial slumber.

Though I worked hard, I tried to make it home early every day to have a catch in the backyard or help with homework. And despite offers of more money to work in New York or L.A., I realized the way to have more was to take less, and the best place to raise a family was at the foot of the Rockies in the tight-knit community of Littleton, Colorado.

Life in Littleton, in fact, seemed to revolve around kids: My family medicine practice was more pediatric than grown-up; I coached Little League baseball, basketball, and football; and I volunteered as the team physician for so many schools, there were days I didn't know who to root for. Life was good and I was content. I had even made peace with my children's grandfather—telling my kids the stories of the good times of my childhood, while leaving out the bad.

Then came two events that shattered my world, and started the wheels that would take me to the ditch.

The first happened in 1999, a seismic blast that shook the country, as well as my life—the Columbine High School shootings. My office was literally a stone's throw from the high school; I knew most of the students, parents, and teachers; and most importantly, of the thirteen who died in the shootings, nine were patients of mine, some of whom I had cared for since the day they were born. And as they fell, so did I.

Soon after, my daughter Katie made history at the University of New Mexico as the first woman ever to play and score points in a major college football game. But her groundbreaking journey was a long and painful one. Katie was originally recruited as a placekicker by the University of Colorado, but a coaching change right before arriving on campus abruptly chilled the atmosphere for a female playing a traditionally all-male sport. It was clear the new head coach, Gary Barnett, didn't want Katie around and a few of the players picked up on the unwelcome message. The harassment started the first day she stepped onto the field, and never let up. She was cursed, groped in the huddle, and had footballs thrown at her head as she practiced her kicking. Soon after the season ended, the nightmare of every father took place: Katie was raped. He was a teammate she considered a friend, the last guy she ever thought would harm her.

It would have been easy to quit, but she never considered it. Katie left Colorado and found a home at the University of New Mexico where she played for a team that accepted and encouraged her to make history. I was proud beyond words the day she trotted onto the field to kick against UCLA on national TV.

She had accomplished her goal, and went on to play in another game the following year at New Mexico. Despite her successes, Katie still had days of darkness, and with them came a struggle I woke to each morning—one inner voice goading me to kill the guy who had raped her while another mocked me as a failure for not protecting her.

My life became a bottomless well of guilt and it seemed the only way to lift myself out was to serve penance: do something to protect, help, *save* the young people of the world. Memories of my dad's experiences resurfaced, and suddenly I knew where I was needed, where I could help, where I might find peace. That place was war. Tonight, though, I wondered if I was just plain stupid: dying in a ditch wasn't going to fix the world or explain the meaning of life.

NOW WE COULD hear whispering and muffled voices in the fields around us. All of the noises were magnified, and my heart thumped like a runaway bass drum. *How long was I in this same spot?* The cramps in my legs answered forever. It was time to move. No one had ever taught me the proper Army techniques of a "low crawl" or "high crawl"; I just slithered along the sandy ground in a way I remembered seeing in war movies. I was surprised at how hard and rocky the ground was; I thought sand was supposed to be soft and friendly, just like at the beach. *Jesus, I miss the beach.* Every year or so we took the kids to Disneyland and the beach in California, but that was the extent of our travels. Not much of an adventurer, I had never even been out of the country until my plane landed in the middle of a war zone just months before.

An odd light caught my attention as I settled into a new position. A red beam from about thirty yards way—it had to be from one of my guys. The beam narrowed to a dot and danced back and forth across my face, then slowly moved to a spot directly over my heart. *Shit, was I a target?* The dot then jerked back and forth from me to the ground. I flattened my body like a pancake into the hard sand.

This time I heard the young sergeant's movement before his voice.

"Sir, you've got to move. You're right between that .50 cal and the hedge. They come through there, your head is going to get blown clear off your neck."

I swung my head around and saw a .50 caliber machine gun on top of a Humvee pointed directly at an opening to the fields. And I was exactly between that opening and the gun. I murmured a sorry and asked where I should go.

"Back to your position, sir. We need you there. Not here."

So much for knowledge of defensive perimeters and tactics. This wasn't what I had in mind when I joined: I was expecting to take care of soldiers, not be one.

WHEN THE WAR erupted in the spring of 2003, the decision to join was far from automatic. I was not some Yankee Doodle doctor who wanted to make the Middle East safe for democracy. I possessed no secret clues about elusive WMDs. And though I loved my country, the start of the conflict didn't infect me with a sudden bout of acute patriotism. But when I heard the Army needed doctors, the deal was clinched. It was all about the kids; maybe not my kids, but someone's kids. Across America were families who went through the motions of life by day and paced the floor by night while their imaginations terrorized their hearts with worry.

So at an age when people retire from the military, I pulled the trigger and became the Army's newest recruit. They even handed me the rank of major, pretty good I was told for a forty-eight-year-old whose military experience consisted of watching *Saving Private Ryan*.

I should have known better. The transition from a comfortable civilian life to instant soldier was my personal version of shock and awe. I was simply too old to enter a world of saluting, marching, or giving orders. And I really *hated* being ordered around, especially when that order was punctuated by a raised voice. I realize a fighting machine isn't built on etiquette, yet I never yelled and expected the same courtesy in return. I got pissed when a pimple-faced instructor more than twenty years my junior called me a "clueless asshole" during basic training. The fatal infraction: a loose thread on the shoulder of my uniform. Christ, the way he screamed you'd have thought I had left a scalpel in him during surgery. When I flicked the thread in his direction and told him a deep, dark anatomical place to stick it, I thought his head would explode. And was disappointed when it didn't.

The brave new world of military courtesy was especially foreign to me: I liked to be called "Dave," not "Sir." Plus, I preferred a "hi" and a handshake when I met someone—a neighborly friendliness that didn't go over very well the first time I met a general. My outstretched hand was greeted with a stunned look, then livid laser beams shooting from his eyes.

Now I caught a whiff of tobacco smoke from beyond the hedge. They were closer. *Would they try to kill us or capture us?* An intelligence briefing said there was a price on our heads—the insurgents were offering cold hard cash for an American taken alive: a captured enlisted soldier was worth $2,500 cash; an officer, $5,000. My crew had made a death pact weeks before during a road trip to Baghdad: we'd fight to the next-to-the-last bullet, then use that last bullet on ourselves to avoid capture—there was simply no way we were going to become stars on an Internet throat-slitting video. As the highest-ranking officer, I would make sure the deeds were done, and then pull the final trigger. I wondered if it would come to that tonight.

THOUGH THE ARMY was quick to snatch me up and start yelling at me, it took more than eight months to get my orders to Iraq. It was January of 2004, less than two weeks before my newly assigned unit departed—and I only got the job because their doctor dropped out at the last minute. Things happened so quickly, there wasn't time to reconsider the leap to war. My kids were torn; on one hand worrying I was going to be shipped home in a casket, on the other, proud I was taking the risk to help soldiers who were, in many cases, the same age as they. We talked a lot about the importance of serving others— being a doer, not just a talker. I hoped I was setting a good example instead of playing the over-the-hill fool.

My new title was "Battalion Surgeon." I was officially attached to the 160th Military Police Airborne Battalion, a reserve unit out of Tallahassee, Florida, which in turn was attached to the 16th MP Airborne Brigade out of Fort Bragg—a unit tasked with security and detainee care around Baghdad and southern Iraq. I was a little confused about where a battalion fit into the scheme of things, but soon found out that their surgeons were typically young, spry, and sharp in military medicine. I was none of the above.

The night I met my new boss, Lieutenant Colonel Izzy Rommes, the first words from his mouth didn't exactly make me feel like a first-round draft pick. After a full thirty seconds of a cold stare from a hard face, he finally drawled, "You sure are one old fucker for this job." Then he stuck his hand out, smiled, and said, "Welcome aboard, Doc. We sure need you, thanks for volunteering."

My new unit quickly took me under their collective wing and led me through the maze of the military, schooling me in the best ways to keep my ass intact. When we arrived in Iraq, their first tasks were to scrounge up scarce body armor, find me an M16 rifle, and make sure

I could shoot it without hitting them, as well as teaching me hand-to-hand combat and self-defense.

The war was quiet when our boots first hit the ground, but within weeks the insurgency came out of hibernation. We were a full eight months from the infamous "Mission Accomplished" moment, now we we had shifted into the "Holy Shit" mode. I spent my deployment carrying an M16 or a shotgun in one hand, medical tools in the other. The months that made up the spring of 2004 were among the bloodiest of the war.

My greeting card to war was a split-second whoosh of air accompanied by stinging shards of glass hitting my face. We were convoying outside Baghdad when someone decided to take a potshot at a moving vehicle. My moving vehicle. We later calculated that the bullet missed my head by little more than an inch. Only weeks before, my biggest enemies in life had been insurance companies who wouldn't approve tests for my patients.

But that was just the beginning. Not only did I get shot at, I was mortared, rocketed, clubbed, and almost stabbed by a group of insurgents, while logging more than two thousand miles convoying the highways and byways of a very pissed-off country. My best stop was Saddam Hussein's palace outside Baghdad; the worst was the infamous Abu Ghraib prison.

The palace was massive and gilded with gold, with the pièce de résistance its bathrooms—beautiful rooms with elegant fixtures and real flush toilets. It had been months since I had had the luxury of using real plumbing, and as I stood over the bowl taking a wicked pee, I pictured Saddam reading the Sunday comics while sitting on the fancy porcelain. Ever so grateful for the facilities, I was even courteous enough to put the seat back down when I was done. But I got a post-pee shiver when I walked over to another structure on the palace grounds—Saddam's so-called party house, a building with a stone etching of Saddam's face on the head of the serpent, handing Eve the apple of sin. The man was truly nuts.

He was also our most famous, and secret, prisoner. Captured a little over a month before my arrival in Iraq, Saddam was hidden away at the High Value Detainee Center at Camp Cropper. As the world was playing a game of "*Where in the World Is Saddam?*", he was right under everyone's nose at a camp in Baghdad just a few miles from the Green Zone. Like many older Iraqi prisoners, this self-proclaimed strongman wasn't very strong when it came to health: Saddam suffered from high blood pressure, a chronic prostate infection, and was the owner of the largest inguinal hernia in the Middle East (which the Army fixed months later). He was also an obsessive neat freak with a fanatical love of Cheetos and Doritos, neither of which helped his blood pressure.

Abu Ghraib was a creepy place filled with ghosts of the tortured. The prison was best known for the detainee abuse that had taken place less than a year before, yet it was hard to ignore the souls of the tens of thousands of Iraqi citizens murdered at the prison by Saddam and his henchmen. The soldiers and marines manning the prison lived in the old cells behind sliding bars. Decorated with American flags and posters, it was impossible to hide the Saddam-era bloodstains on the walls or the hooks once used as tools of torture. Whenever our unit stopped at Abu, I begged off the offer of a guest cell, choosing instead to sleep under the chassis of a truck parked in the courtyard. It wasn't the most comfortable place to spend the night, especially when a rocket landed and bounced me into the undercarriage, but it was still better than sleeping inside the house of horror.

THE EXOTIC VOICES from the fields were getting louder. Too many voices. I took a quick look at the fuel trucks, knowing they'd be hit first, and wondered if I'd get a shot off before being burned to a crisp. Whispered orders made their way among us. Lock and load. Safeties off. Here we go. I thought of my family, my dad, my stupidity. *Had I really accomplished anything?* Without warning, a growling thunder erupted from down the road, steadily overtaking the noises from the hedge. The ground began to shake and I thought my world was coming to an end. I was wrong. While it wasn't a true John Wayne moment with gunshots and fireworks, it was John Wayne enough for me. Our cavalry came rumbling to the rescue: a half a dozen heavily armed gun trucks with a massive tow truck bringing up the rear. We cautiously got up and moved toward our rescuers, grins of relief splitting our faces. I was scheduled to go home in three days and now it looked like I'd live to make the trip.

THE CONVERSATION WITH my dad that night took place in bits and pieces over the course of three long hours, more time than I had with him on the ride to Philly. The words were never spoken aloud, yet I felt sure that he knew that I had just learned his bitter lesson of war: fear. Sure, I was scared of dying—it's hard not to think that way when you are lying in the dark . . . waiting.

But worse was the fear of leaving my loved ones behind and the pain they would feel with my death. Then came the fear of screwing up and causing the deaths of my fellow soldiers. Unforgivable.

As I walked with shaking legs to my Humvee with my wiry young sergeant, I apologized repeatedly for screwing up as we'd hid for our lives in the ditch.

"Hell, I didn't know what I was doing back there. I could have gotten us all killed. Man, I am so sorry."

It wasn't until our Humvee was headed toward the safety of our base that it hit me, three long decades after a car ride down the Jersey Turnpike. The young sergeant had answered with a smile and quick thumbs-up.

WHICH END
DO THE BULLETS COME OUT?

THE FIRST CASUALTY of the deployment took place eight thousand miles away from the war zone. I was tiptoeing and stumbling around in the dark at three in the morning, making sure I had packed all the civilian luxuries necessary to survive life in the desert when I rammed my little toe into the edge of the couch. A few curse words went flying, along with two huge armfuls of nonmilitary essentials such as an iPod, laptop, razors, toilet paper, and a mini-library of paperbacks. I silently gathered up the scattered pile, hoping the computer and the toe weren't broken, then limped outside and sat in cool predawn air, taking in the sweetness of the freshly mown lawn whose blades I had trimmed the night before. No yard to worry about for a while—instead of crabgrass, I'd be battling dust and sand.

It had been three years since my tour in Iraq, and the war continued to go badly. The Army still needed warm bodies to fill its medical needs, but since I had already done time in the "Sandbox," they offered me a comfortable stateside slot doing routine physicals. I turned them down flat. It wasn't bravery or bravado; I simply needed to go back. I wish I could explain why. And my family wished I could explain why. They'd been through hell during my last deployment, especially after seeing pictures of me cradling a rifle. This time, I assured them, I'd be safer. I had grabbed an assignment to a CSH, or combat support hospital, today's equivalent of a Mobile Army Surgical Hospital, or MASH. No more rifles; no more convoys; no more face time with crazed insurgents.

The nature of the war had changed, with IEDs becoming the conflict's four-letter word. Just thinking of an Improvised Explosive Device sent shivers up my spine; we'd dealt with them in 2004, but the ones hidden on the roads these days packed a more powerful punch, enough to blow a five-ton truck ten feet into the air. I simply didn't want to picture what something that violent would do to a delicate human body, but would soon find out. From what I had been told, we'd see fewer gunshot wounds and more blown-up bodies. A voice on the phone from Medical Corps Headquarters said, "Be ready, Major, business will be booming." The horrible play on words made me grimace.

The truth was I would be busy. The timing of my deployment meant I had volunteered to be a part of the next great military campaign that sounded suspiciously like an energy drink: "The Surge." I didn't know what exactly I was getting into, but at least this time I'd be with a group of doctors rather than running around with a bunch of young, savvy combat troops. I prayed my new colleagues would be capable and easy to work with, but I wasn't overly hopeful. Doctors, as a rule, tend to be big on ego, short on social skills.

As I put my feet up on a lawn chair, my mind wandered back to the office and the last patients of the previous day, one an overweight smoker with diabetes who couldn't find time to exercise because he was too busy. But he was remembering to take his medicine . . . most days. *Hell, man*, I thought, *I'm going to war tomorrow to take care of people who don't have choices about their health—you do.* Yet I simply shook his hand and told him to keep up the good work . . . *and please try not to drop dead before I get back.*

The other patient on my worry list was a four-year-old with a fever and an ear infection. He seemed a little more listless than he should have been. Maybe I should have done some tests. Maybe I was just fretting like a grandmother. Either way, I wondered if people realize how often we doctors worried about the decisions we made, carrying our worries home to spend the night. Maybe I could call from Fort Benning later and find out how the kid was doing.

I watched my wristwatch sweep away the minutes—cursing it for not hurrying so I could get my journey started, yet at the same time swearing at it for racing too rapidly. As the sun peeked over the horizon and reflected against the foothills of the Rockies, I realized I was lonely and scared, and hadn't even left my driveway. My orders didn't say exactly where I was headed; simply IRAQ in small letters— as if I wouldn't notice—but the grapevine hinted my destination was going to be some ramshackle combat hospital near Tikrit, home-town of Iraq's favorite son, Saddam Hussein. My new unit would be the 399th CSH.

The neighbor's dog trotted over and smeared a good-luck slobber across my face, then promptly turned and scooted across to a nice green patch of turf, where he squatted and dropped a big turd. All I could hope was that his steamy dump wasn't an omen.

We decided the whole family would drive me to the airport and attempt to perform an artificially cheery goodbye. Then I'd head off east while they'd head back for a family breakfast, all of us pretending the next few months would speed by like a meteor.

The flight from Denver to Atlanta was a quick one—too quick as I thought about how I would spend the next several months in a life foreign to what I had lived for five decades. Instead of privacy, I would spend every hour surrounded and suffocated by others—in a noisy, chaotic, and often bloody environment. Toeing the line, salut-ing, acting like an officer, and making sure my monotonous uniform fit proper regulations—with no loose threads. No matter how hard I tried, I still had trouble adjusting to the fact I was a soldier.

I reached into my back pocket and pulled out, after my official orders, the most important papers I would carry this deployment: my dad's wallet and logbook from his days in World War II. I read the names of the men he commanded: White, Murphy, Kuel, Rizzi, Stein—more than three dozen in all—and wondered how they, and their families, felt on the day in 1943 when they reported to duty, especially the ones whose names my dad had crossed out by a single line. These were young men who died in combat, and in small letters next to their crossed-out names and lives were the penciled-in names of their replacements. Some of those names wound up being split by a pencil stroke, too.

World War II was the "good war," but I wondered just how good it was to those families who received the dreaded telegram from the War Department, saying their husband, son, or brother wouldn't be coming home. And now more than fifty years later had still not come home. How was life for those families in the decades since? And how would life be for the families of the more than four thousand Americans who wouldn't be coming home from my war? Could I and would I make a difference? My mind and heart argued the question. I thrust the thoughts and numbers from my brain, wondering as my plane began its descent whether I was equipped to prevent any more patriotic deaths in a controversial war.

In Atlanta, I made my way to the connecting gate to Columbus, home of Fort Benning, where my father had spent the first months of his war attending infantry and officer candidate school.

At the gate, I caught more than a few soldiers staring at me. Most were sharply dressed in creased and pressed battle uniforms and there I was, slouching against a wall in faded jeans and T-shirt—a pretty cool T-shirt actually, with a silk-screened picture of a surfboard cutting through a curling wave. *Oh man, here we go.* I didn't need a bunch of hard-asses giving me *the look.* Worse, what if the gawkers were the doctors I'd be working with? Shit. I needed relaxed, not rigid. Pranksters, not pricks. As we boarded our puddle jumper for the flight down the road to Columbus, all I could think of was how I could survive life with a bunch of industrial-strength douche bags for the next four months.

The first thing to hit me when we landed at the small Columbus airport was the thick Georgia humidity, the second was the piercing screech of a wide-brimmed sergeant yelling for everyone to get on the buses after grabbing our bags.

"How quick we leaving?" I asked.

"Quick. Real quick." He scowled.

"I gotta pee, Sarge."

"Make it quick. Real quick. Buses wait for no one."

Big Hat finished his sentence with a face-shattering grimace, but since I wasn't in uniform, he didn't know whether to yell at me or play it safe and treat me like an officer. My advanced age probably tipped the scales toward courtesy.

One empty and happy bladder later, I left the bathroom and was met with an "Are you by any chance a doctor . . . uh, sir?"

Big Hat must have figured an unkempt, shuffling guy like me could be nothing but a doctor, and his tone downshifted from gruff to soft when I answered a wholehearted "Yup."

"Sir, please hustle out to bus number two, that's the bus for the medical people. If you need a hand with your duffel I can rustle up some help."

I grinned and said thanks, I could handle my gear by myself, and I solemnly promised I would go straight to bus number 2 and not wander off and get lost.

"We roll out in three minutes, sir."

In typical Army efficiency, bus number 2 didn't roll out in three minutes, five minutes, or even fifteen minutes. An hour was more like it, with forty of us getting to be closer friends than we wanted, sitting on top of each other in a muggy vehicle built for twenty-four. As I swung my head around scanning the bus, I realized everyone wore jeans and casual clothes. No starched or even unstarched uniforms in sight. Thank you, Jesus.

On half of my lap was an older blond, brush-cut guy who told me he was from Okinawa . . . or was it Oshkosh? After seeing my confusion, someone who knew him spoke up from the row behind and translated.

He said Oklahoma.

"Oh. Nice to meet you. Dave Hnida from Colorado. Family doc."

"Rick Reutlinger, Muskogee, Oklahoma. Surgeon."

"Isn't that a song or something?"

"You bet, the 'Okie from Muskogee,' by Merle Haggerty."

Haggerty? I'd heard of Merle Haggard . . .

"So, Rick, where you headed?"

"Tikrit."

"Me, too. How many of us are there?"

"I think eight docs. But have no idea who the hell all these other people are that are trying to feel each other up on this damned bus. They're all medical people but headed someplace else. Sorry about my ass, by the way."

"No problem. It's nice and soft."

"Fat and spongy is more like it."

I learned Rick Reutlinger had never been to Iraq but had served a tour in Afghanistan in late 2004. He spoke in a rapid-fire drawl—I only understood about half of what he said, but was able to decipher that, besides being a general surgeon, he was a huge Texas A&M fan, had been a veterinarian before going to medical school, owned a farm, and drove a pickup truck. A bus of sardined soldiers had given me a chance introduction to the mumble-mouth surgeon who would go on to be my colleague, cheerleader . . . and most importantly, my best friend during the next four months.

As the rust-coated bus chugged along I-185 doing a rickety 30 mph, I stared out the window at the thick Georgia pines, grateful to have made a buddy so quickly, and hoping the rest of my group would be just as friendly. I didn't realize at the time some of the men on this bus would go on to become the best friends I'd ever had.

We were deposited in front of the CRC, otherwise known as the CONUS Replacement Center, a cluster of World War II–era concrete buildings painted a nauseating shade of sinus infection yellow. We lined up in a formation that looked like an incomplete jigsaw puzzle, and were told to wait for the rest of the people who would be joining us to train for our mission overseas. With our small group, we calculated we could blow through the process and be on our way in a day or two. Then we heard our delay before we saw it: more than 350 civilian contractors who would swallow us up and slow us down. They came from everywhere, scurrying in a confused frenzy like someone had just stomped their anthill.

The Army called it a Charlie Foxtrot—or Cluster Fuck—and in this case, I couldn't think of a better term. Why in hell's name were we training with a bunch of civilians, many of whom would staff the PXs, run the laundries, and supervise food services? It took twenty minutes to get everyone into some semblance of a formation.

We were told we had six days at Benning to get ready for our mission before boarding a flight to Iraq—and sorry, but tough shit, with the Surge we're running more people through than ever. We medical folks stole quick glances at each other and murmured a few curses. Hell, we shouldn't have been surprised—not only were we rapidly sending over tens of thousands of troops, we also needed tens of thousands of civilians who would do the jobs soldiers used to do: cook, clean, run recreation facilities, and make sure the laundry got done. And the American contingent would do pretty well for a year's work: 50–150 grand—all tax-free.

How times had changed. In World War II, the percentage of contractors to military was 3 percent; Korea 5 percent; Vietnam and the Gulf War saw the number rise to 10 percent. Now with the number of soldiers vaulting to 180,000 in the months to come, the percentage of contractors would hit an identical number—a 50-50 split. Many weren't even well-paid Americans; it seems we hired a lot of Iraqis, Sri Lankans, Russians, and other "third country nationals" to do the menial work that paid them what would be pauper's wages in America—but big bucks in their home countries. Talk about the privatization of war.

The gun to start the race to deploy was fired quickly. Our bloated group was herded, then stuffed like sausages into a hot tent and cooked until overdone. We were subjected to hours of death by PowerPoint on subjects such as: "Be nice to your fellow soldier" and "Don't get an STD." We were also given crash courses on the climate in the Middle East (a little helpful), Middle Eastern culture (a little less helpful), and how to pull guard duty (to which I thought, if I'm pulling guard duty, the war is lost).

The only amusement of the day came when we were fed lunch, one MRE per person, with exactly enough Meals Ready to Eat for each person—no seconds, no extras. Our famished group lumbered up a small hill and plucked the plastic bags containing our meals out of the back of a drab green cargo truck, but some slippery fingers left me with an empty stomach.

"Dave, where's your food, dude?" It was Bill Stanton, our newly met orthopedist who was also Tikrit-bound—and seemed like a friendly guy . . .

Rick answered for me. "Listen to this. So me and Dave grab our MRE things and figure it's a good idea to hit the porta-johns before eating. I'm next door peeing when I hear this pinball machine next door. Ping-ping-ping-ping. Then a loud splash . . . then an even louder "Shit!" Turns out we had one MRE bouncing off the walls and now floating in a sea of blue-coated turds."

"Dude, I hope you stitch better than you piss."

Bill laughed.

Both Ricky and Bill then dug through their extras and made sure I at least had something to quiet my stomach. It was the first of many emergency meals they would serve me that summer.

The war against hunger didn't get much better on day two. Up at 5 A.M., we trudged to the mess tent where we were greeted by a not-so-cheery bunch of civilians standing behind a steam table doling out breakfast.

I held my flimsy plastic plate up like a begging child.

"I'll take the scrambled eggs, pancakes, and a couple slices of bacon, please."

"One entrée and one side." Scowling, she didn't give me much time to make a choice.

The server next to her chimed in.

"So what's it going to be? Keep the line moving or get out."

"What's a side? The bacon? Potatoes? That gray stuff moving on its own?"

Another cold hard stare.

Well, I guess you're not morning people, are you?

"Okay, fill me up with whatever isn't against the law."

One small scoop of rock-hard scrambled eggs and one thin slice of fat impersonating bacon plopped onto my plate.

Rick stared at my tray, particles of imitation eggs stuck to the corners of his mouth.

"That's one deadly coronary artery plaque right there, Davy-boy. That's if the food servers don't kill you first."

Rick's quip was washed down with a lukewarm cup of watery coffee mixed with paint thinner. Sons of bitches. I was a coffee addict, and you would think the Army would be coffee experts. Not even close. It reminded me of the sorry days during my first deployment when I would simply spoon out and swallow granules of Taster's Choice whenever we were on the road and I needed to wake up after a short night's sleep.

My stomach was still growling as we lined up for yet another formation—and got a mandatory chewing out for a variety of offenses, real and imagined.

"You people need to step it up a notch. Our EDD is now five

days. Your LO for the day is gear, then you'll head for FAC and issues about EPW at the ROC. Remember we're just a MAT for you people and we need your help. Your POC is Sergeant Smith if you have questions."

Holy smokes! What was that alphabet soup of instructions? I felt like I needed to watch "Army Sesame Street" so I could decipher the acronyms.

I turned to Rick.

"Did you get any of that?"

"Nope, but I think we showed up at the wrong army. That's Chinese or something coming out of that guy's mouth. Well, let's just follow everybody else, like always."

We stood still as the massive formation dissolved into small groups and finally spotted a few of the doctors collecting near a doorway. We headed in that direction and soon were bused over to an acronym that I knew, the CIF or Central Issue Facility—a giant three-block-long dull brick warehouse bursting with equipment. We were handed four duffel bags in which to stuff five duffels' worth of gear including Kevlar helmet, body armor, mosquito netting, and the all-important shovel and entrenching tool—what I was going to shovel and entrench at a hospital, I didn't know.

Three hours later, we thought we had everything we could possibly need—until we hit the last station where we were issued winter jackets, fleece parkas, long underwear, and cold weather gloves. We were now officially set for a trip to Antarctica, where to the best of our knowledge, there were no active ongoing combat operations.

Later that day we were issued our weapons, an M9 automatic handgun. Veterans mockingly called it the popgun, yet it was better than throwing stones . . . a little. Popgun or not, it was a valuable, and expensive, weapon being placed in our care. For the rest of the week, every time I went into the porta-john—aka the blue canoe—I held on to that pistol like it was a million-dollar winning lottery ticket. Drop that baby into the blue canoe and I'd have to go fishing.

That night we sat in our cramped room assembling gear—stuffing heavy armor plates into the lining of the combat vest, and trying on uniforms, which came in the two standard Army sizes, too large and too small. As I surveyed four duffelsful of junk dumped on the floor, I realized we were now an army of Velcro. Grenade pouches, ammo holders, and holsters were all attached by Velcro instead of snaps. I had Rick help attach my Velcro helmet liner and webbing since I had no clue which tab stuck to which. At one point my helmet Velcro got stuck on my crotch Velcro and I couldn't pull it loose. Some guy walking by our open door looked stunned as he watched me frantically pull, yank, and punch at my helmeted groin.

An experienced soldier could have assembled everything in thirty minutes; it took me more than four hours, even with help. But even then, I wasn't done—it all had to be stuffed back into the duffels. That exercise turned into a game of mulligans and do-overs: fill up the bags—then, in anger, kick the leftovers still on the floor—dump the bags, then try different combinations in different duffels. It was like a game show, guessing what would fit where. I finally fell asleep one pissed-off civilian in an Army costume.

We were greeted the next morning by a foul-looking breakfast of some dark, shiny material dumped on top of a stone-hard biscuit (Rick swore it looked like something he removed from an old lady the week before), then headed out to the morning's formation. It was scheduled for 0600, but Rick scurried at a pace worthy of an Olympic race walker.

As he puffed up a small incline he said, "If you're not ten minutes early, you're five minutes late." It was the debut of a phrase that would attack me every morning in the months to come. I was joined at the hip to a new best friend—but a new best friend who was also an obsessive, anal-compulsive surgeon who loved to be early. It was a sharp contrast to my "the war will still be there when we get there" attitude. But since he helped me with the major construction project called my equipment the night before, I was obligated to scurry along like a kid late for school.

We arrived before the rest of the crew, which turned out to be a great way to attach names to the faces of the people we would be working with—I had met everyone the first day yet still mixed up names and jobs. The obsessive-compulsive Rick was like human Directory Assistance as the docs made their way up the small hill.

"Now, you know Billy Stanton, right? Ortho. He's from Florida. That big black guy with the giant muscles is another surgeon. Bernard Harrison. Nice fella. Minnesota.

"Mike Barron is like you. A family doc who is supposed to work in the ER. The flat head comes from him being an ex-marine. From St. Louis.

"The husky one with big glasses is the other ER guy, Gerry Maloney. I think from Ohio. The short guy behind him is our other surgeon—Ian Nunnally. He's from Ohio, too. Kind of quiet. The older guy with the gray hair yapping away is Colonel Blok—anesthesia gas passer from I don't where. Then all of those others, hell, I think they're doctors or anesthetists or something. But they ain't going to Tikrit. I just heard they'll train with us this week."

Close to forty in all, only eight of us were doctors who would head off to staff a little hospital sitting smack in the middle of the Surge.

As others fell into formation, we murmured his and good mornings. Except for Billy, who already knew Rick's obsession with the clock.

"Dudes, when did you guys get here, last night?"

His answer was an interruption from the front of the formation, a squealing "We're still not getting done fast enough, people—what's wrong with us?"

Hell, we didn't know what was wrong with us, and I don't think we really cared, but we did learn we were heading over to "Medical" to make sure we were fit enough to deploy.

We all thought it common sense the medical screening would

be the most thorough of all the things we did that week. After all, you wouldn't want to send a soldier with a hidden medical condition off to the war zone. It turned out the screening did wind up taking a lot of time, but it was anything but thorough. Out of the four hours we spent at the medical station, a grand eight minutes was spent on actual screening. The essentials included making sure our vaccinations were up to date, we weren't carrying HIV in our blood, and that we could hear little toots and beeps in a soundproof booth. My shots were still good from my last deployment, my rapid HIV was negative, and my hearing test was a pass. Then it was my turn for a face-to-face meeting with the physician: How are you feeling? Okay. Any medical problems not listed on the form? No. Great, you're good to go, and thanks for serving our country.

No blood pressure check. No listening to my heart. No vision test. Not even a hand in front of the face and guessing how many fingers I could see. As far as the Army was concerned, I was good to go.

But Rick wasn't. He had failed his hearing test—badly—and needed an MRI of his head before deploying. The test was scheduled at 9 A.M. the next day, so he'd miss the fun of a group of forty doctors and anesthetists playing soldier, the big event on the schedule of day three at Benning. It was a day that would highlight our cluelessness.

Out on the makeshift training grounds, we shimmied under and caught our pants on barbed wire, pushed the overweight docs by their butts over not-so-Himalayan three-foot walls, and threw fake hand grenades, which more times than not hit the instructors rather than the targets.

We then were sent to an adjacent field, handed dummy M16 rifles, and practiced turning and firing from different postures and positions. We were all supposed to turn in the same direction, then rapid-fire a series of blanks. Sounds easy . . . except for a group of civilian doctors. Typically, half of the group spun one way, the other half the other, and we wound up blasting each other with surprised wide-eyed looks painted on our faces. The only true casualty was one doc who bloodied his lip bringing his weapon to the ready position as we sidestepped down a make-believe alley in a wide-open grassy field. ("Use your imagination, people!")

The afternoon, however, brought a true adventure in terror: taking our M9 pistols apart and cleaning them. Some of the younger doctors had never handled a weapon before, and since we were given no formal instruction all we could do was try to help each other out was offer a few words of encouragement as the instructors raced through our section of the tent.

The M9 pistol has a thick, dangerous spring hidden deep inside, and before you could say "Incoming," there were springs rocketing like missiles through the tent, striking people in the head, face, and neck. We could only hope the remaining two days would be casualty-free.

The following morning started with a smattering of catch-up paperwork, followed by a mandatory course on first-aid. Mandatory meant *everyone*, even physicians.

The instructor stood with his hands on his hips as he blared instructions in a wailing monotone.

"If someone's bleeding, what's the best way to take care of it? You put pressure on it, people. And if someone's in shock, elevate their legs above the level of their heart. Then wait for the experts. It's not that difficult, people."

Our eyes rolled like bowling balls. Thanks for the instruction, I was sure we were heading over to Iraq because they needed doctors to elevate legs, then call for help. *People.*

The final task was to qualify with our pistols, meaning we had to hit a certain number of targets before we'd be allowed in hostile territory with a loaded weapon. The course was a series of plastic targets that sprung up in a random sequence at distances of anywhere from ten to fifty meters. I thought the green targets were shaped like little Iraqi women in robes, which was a little freakish. When my turn came up, I walked down the firing line with a group of ten other shooters and punched a magazine of ammo into my pistol. At the order of "Fire," the first "little woman" sprung up and with it a sensation of being in the middle of a bag of microwaving popcorn. Pop-pop-pop. But while my body was holding my weapon at Benning, my mind was in Iraq. In 2004. Outside Baghdad. And the pops were real gunfire. I just stared at the first several targets as they sprung up, then down—I was unable to squeeze off a single shot. Then just as suddenly, the time machine dropped me back at Benning—and I hit the next thirty silhouettes in a row. Sharpshooter. Not bad for a doctor. But I had never frozen in any situation before. Bad for a doctor. *What the hell happened? And would it happen again?*

That night, we sat on the grass and drank our one-night-only treat of a final beer, celebrating the news that Rick was medically cleared and able to deploy with the group. We had already started to bond as a team, and worry over our ability to work together slowly dissolved. The only thing left was the anxiety over how I personally would perform.

As I tossed and turned in my bunk that final night, I flashed back to a time more than sixty years earlier . . . My dad had spent his nights at Benning with a flashlight under his covers—surviving on an hour or two of sleep as he studied for officer training—afraid he would wash out or miss an important point that might cost a life in war outside a lesson plan. How would I do? Did I know enough? Would I freeze? A part of me dreaded the answers. It made no sense; I'd already been in the war and didn't run away, but this time was different. I'd be on the other side of the helicopter; instead of sending wounded to the experts, I was supposed to be the expert saving them.

The next morning we bused to the airport and were stuffed into a plane that was retired from commercial service in the 1970s, and before entering the cockpit, the pilot went from soldier to soldier thanking each for our service. I thought it was a nice gesture, until it was time for takeoff and he got on the intercom saying, "Don't you listen to what the media has to say. We are going to win this war. Ignore CNN, the Communist News Network."

Shit, I didn't need a lunatic flying us over the ocean in a duct-taped aircraft. But at least I was stuffed into a middle seat between two overweight contractors who would provide great padding if we crashed.

CAMP BORING

IT TOOK EIGHTEEN hours for DTA, or Duct-Taped Airlines, to deliver us to the Promised Land. The good news: the flight was free. The bad: I drew the middle seat for the marathon journey and was surrounded by the enemy for a nonstop nightmare. Such as the guy who sat in the row in front of me, you know, the one who cranks his seat back until your knees greet your throat. In the window seat was a rustic fellow who decided it was okay to chew tobacco as long as he spat its tarlike residue into a handheld paper cup. The problem, though, was a mouth with the aim of a drunken garden hose. I watched stringy lines of black goo fly onto my uniform and coalesce into the solid patches of a malodorous pothole repair. As I dodged the liquid bullets from the left of me, I was trying to figure out why the guy to the right of me smelled like a commercial for lactose intolerance. It suddenly struck me six hours into the flight—a momentous revelation, in fact—that the Army did this on purpose to make soldiers *want* to get to Iraq.

Blessed respite and fresh air came with a short fuel stop in Budapest. It was mid-afternoon local time and we were allowed to wander

the crowded concourse for the one-hour refueling. Rick and I meandered through the terminal, watching the locals scurry to board flights
to wherever Hungarians travel. As we watched them, they watched
us—a huge mass of American soldiers in uniform strolling through
their airport—and gave us a wide berth, pulling their gawking children out of the way. Although we were now allies, it seemed the old-
est Hungarians stared at us as if we were Germans or Russians from
decades past. We grabbed a sandwich and a Coke, snapped some
pictures, and generally wasted time walking cramps out of our legs.

We landed in the furnace known as Kuwait City shortly before
midnight and were quickly herded onto buses for a quick trip to Camp
Buehring, the usual stopover for troops heading into Iraq. It was a
time for soldiers fresh from the States to adjust body clocks as well as
to the scorching temperatures of the Middle East. But I don't know if
anyone truly acclimated to the heat, you simply suffered through it as
you waited for the oven timer to ring at the end of your deployment.
Although our watches said 11 P.M., our bodies said 9 A.M. and our
brains said . . . nothing. The Army could have flown us the long way
to Kansas City for all we knew. The group was deathly quiet as many
wiped the dribble of openmouthed sleep onto their sleeves while stag-
gering in a semidrunken line toward the waiting vehicles. I held on to
the back of Rick's uniform as he put his hand on the person in front
of him and so forth all the way up to the front of the line. We looked
like a group of preschoolers on a field trip as we shuffled to the buses.
Those who managed to take in the surroundings mumbled disappointment. Far from looking like a war zone, Kuwait International Airport
was a mirror image of every major airport in America.

We slid into our seats and a few tried to steal a glance at the scen-
ery as we pulled away, but the interior of the bus was dark and there
were thick curtains over the windows—supposedly to keep anyone
with evil intentions from seeing a bus filled with arriving American
troops. But as our wheels rolled along the modern superhighway,
I couldn't help but wonder why someone with a bomb or rocket-

propelled grenade—as well as half a brain—couldn't just add it all up as a juicy target. We might as well have had banners with big letters and flashing lights on the side of the locally chartered bus proclaiming: "Welcome to Kuwait! Thanks for saving our asses in 1991."

The trip from Kuwait International to our next stop, Camp Buehring, was forty miles—thirty-eight on paved highway, then two more across the surface of the moon, craters and all. A dark potholed dirt road, which we traversed at about 4 mph. We slammed into each other with each bump and at one point heard a warning scream from the back of the bus about an overripe bladder ready to burst with the next jolt. We weren't given the chance to urinate as we transitioned from plane to bus to Buehring. Lesson learned: pee whenever you can, wherever you can—even in front of a group of people. The Army couldn't care less about your urinary tract.

We finally pulled up to the gate at 3 A.M. where a spry, full-bird colonel jumped on board. Sporting a big dark battle patch on his sleeve with slanted white stripes, he belonged to the 3rd Infantry Division and needed to hitch a ride onto the base. As the colonel grabbed a seat up front, someone spied the patch and groggily mumbled, "3rd Infantry," to which the fully awake colonel jumped up and screamed the 3rd ID's slogan, which dated back to World War I: "ROCK OF THE MARNE!" Rick had been sleeping soundly on my shoulder and the battle cry startled and confused him.

"What did he say? Top of the morning?"

I stifled a laugh. "No, Ricky, Rock of the Marne."

"That's what I said. Top of the morning. That's nice of him but man, it's late."

"No, Rick. Rock—of—the—Marne. Go back to sleep."

"Which *Rocky* movie was that? Three or Four?"

With that, I bit off a loud laugh and now had the eyes of one pissed-off colonel centered on my face. I was punchy with a severe case of the giggles and waiting for the teacher at the front of the classroom to yell at me.

"No, Ricky, it was *Rocky Ten*, where he beats the shit out of the Nazis."

"He didn't fight the Nazis."

More clipped bursts of stifled laughter.

"Yes he did, it was the one where he dumped Adrian for Eva Braun at the end."

"Oh. Missed that one."

"Major, you got a problem back there?" Colonel Marne had steam coming out of his ears and was staring at us like misbehaving school kids.

"Ah, no, sir. My buddy here and me, uh, we were just telling some stories."

"Well, shape up! You're in theater now." *Meaning the war zone. No laughing allowed.*

"Roger that, sir, and by the way, top of the morning to you."

Now wide awake, Rick almost peed his pants laughing. The colonel shook his head. "You're a bunch of damned doctors, aren't you?"

"Yes, sir, just looking for the golf course."

Buehring was a dump—its soil hard as concrete with about an inch of fine powdery sand on top, every step morphed into a walk on the moon, leaving astronaut footprints behind. The air was hot and filled with fine particles that we inhaled with every breath. Someone complained about the baritone hum and thumping of the ever-present generators that powered lights that made 4 A.M. seem like high noon. It was a noise that would follow us the rest of our deployment. The bright lights didn't scare away the cat-sized kangaroo rats that roamed the camp, and I was a little freaked about the deadly desert vipers that had a reputation for slithering into porta-johns. I was now paranoid to sit on the pot and have something sink its fangs into my dangling parts.

We finally bedded down at about 4:30 in a cavernous Quonset-type tent. It seemed like there were hundreds of these identical white huts lined up. To play it safe, I wrote the number of our hut in ink on my wrist so I wouldn't wander into the wrong one, day or night. After forming a human conveyor belt, we passed our overstuffed duffels down the line and dumped them into a big pile in the middle of the giant tent, then collapsed in a heap—asleep within seconds.

The tent was bare-bones, the cots sand- and dust-covered, with our body armor used as makeshift pillows. Most of us woke less than an hour later; I was shaking violently and had icicles on my mustache. Too hot outside, now too cold inside—the air conditioner had been preset to subarctic temperatures. In the dark, I dug through my gear, pulling out my sleeping bags, extra uniform gloves, and some of the winter gear we'd been issued at Benning. I shivered my way back to sleep, sucking in frozen dust particles with each breath.

As the days crawled by, we renamed our camp from Buehring to Boring. It was clear we were just wasting time until we could catch a flight into Tikrit. A slow depression began to sink into the group— the weather was suffocating with temperatures tickling the 120 mark, that is, until we trudged back to our subzero tent for a frigid night of shaking and shimmying. Instead of clear desert skies, we baked under an ominous dark gray overcast, which at times opened up and angrily pelted us with large globs of muddy rain. The food sucked, and to squander time, we were forced to endure lecture after lecture on subjects such as first-aid (make sure you elevate the legs!) and IEDs (don't step on them, they're bad!), and suffer through training sessions on the military computer system of the future, which meant we wouldn't be using it this deployment.

Our only good day at Boring included an hour-long, kidney-bruising bus ride to the firing range located somewhere out in the middle of Nowhere, Kuwait, where we needed to pop in and fire a clip of ammo to make sure our weapons had survived the long journey over the ocean. The quick session produced no jams, no misdirected shots, and best of all, no springs flying through the air looking for a face to lacerate.

For a lot of the group, the trip was a scenic wonderland—they'd never seen the endless desert of the Middle East or the Bedouins who inhabited it. *Look at those camels, man. Very cool.* I'd had my fill of sandy landscape from the thousands of convoy miles logged my last trip—yet still looked out and stared at the Bedouins, simple people who spent their entire lives moving from place to place in the desert. I wondered how much they knew or even cared about this war—this conflict was probably just one more through the centuries they and their ancestors tried to avoid.

After firing, we returned to the camp for more lectures, and were told we'd now be busing to a different base, where we'd actually catch our flight into Iraq. Once again, we underwent the drill of packing, dragging, lugging, and finally forming a fire bucket brigade to get our obese duffel bags into our new home at Camp Ali Al Saleem. Here the accommodations were anything but cavernous; our bunk beds touched, and as a group we had to decide the best direction to sleep to avoid shoving our reeking feet under the nose of the guy in the next bunk.

Buehring was an amusement park compared to Al Saleem; there wasn't much to do except wait in an endless line for a fifteen-minute Internet slot or a quick phone call to home. Even the thrill of some fast food from the Golden Arches, nicknamed "McArab's" because of its Arabic signage, didn't last more than a few happy meals. But our boredom had one saving grace; we finally had the time to get to know each other a little better.

My buddy since day one on the bus at Benning was the fifty-four-year-old clean-shaven, disciplined conformist from a rural and conservative part of Oklahoma. Rick Reutlinger's uniform always looked sharp, he had perfected a snappy salute, and was always respectful of his superiors. In other words, everything I was not. But a long summer together would give me a chance to corrupt him.

Bernard Harrison was a handsome, debonair heart surgeon from Minneapolis. He even had a slick pencil-thin mustache that added an air of suave. Prim and proper, the name "Bernard" fit him perfectly, which made it a slam dunk to christen him "Harry" instead. He was forty-nine, single, and had the chiseled body of a stud twenty years younger. The women would love him when we got to Tikrit.

Our third surgeon was thirty-five-year-old Ian Nunnally, the youngest of the group. Known as "Little Buddha," Ian had served as an enlisted soldier more than a decade before, so he knew his way around the military. Fresh from residency, Ian was quiet as we started our journey and we hoped he'd loosen up over time. We didn't know if it was worry over the war, us, or something else.

Our bone man was a square-jawed forty-four-year-old orthopedist named Bill Stanton from Fort Pierce, Florida. "Wild Bill" was regular Army for years and had served in places like Kosovo before leaving the military and going into private practice. He rejoined after 9/11 and asked to be sent to the war. Bill was a graduate of West Point and wore the huge ring of the military academy. He had the easy look of someone's older brother; I felt like I'd known him for years.

Mike Barron, the family doctor from St. Louis, was slated to work with me in the ER. Mike was an infantry officer in the Marines, then performed an abrupt about-face leaving the Corps and going off to medical school. He was on the faculty of the St. Louis University School of Medicine and now hoped to go out and medically minister to the Iraqi civilian population as well as our own wounded.

We couldn't quite get a handle on our other ER doc, Gerry Maloney. In the real world, Gerry was a thirty-eight-year-old toxicologist who was smart as hell and *loved* the Army. Or at least loved the *idea* of the Army and its unique language. A conversation with Gerry usually consisted of mil-language with a touch of reality sprinkled in.

When Rick and I would run into Gerry, we'd ask, "What's shaking, babe?"

"Zulu."

"What the hell is Zulu?"

"Zulu. Zero. Nothing. C'mon, guys, it's SOP to know the lingo. You'll need it once those air jockeys get us in country."

Despite the heavy doses of "Maloney baloney," we loved Gerry and decided the best way to handle him would be to adopt him as our group mascot. "Gerry, you are an Alpha Sierra Sierra, but you're *our* Alpha Sierra Sierra."

The doctor with the highest military rank was a crusty character we called Charlie Brown, an affectionate nickname that evolved from his real name of Robert Blok to Blockhead to Charlie Brown. Charlie was a full-bird colonel, one step below general. He seemed to know every rule and regulation ever invented by the Army, including the recommended distance from tent to latrine. I'm sure he even counted the steps. He was our anesthesiologist, and was in charge of a group of four nurse anesthetists who would accompany us to the CSH, the combat support hospital.

As we talked, I discovered I had the least amount of military experience in the group, a relative baby with just over three years in the service. But I did have one bit of priceless experience none of the others did—combat. I didn't know what the conditions would be like when we finally got into Iraq, but I knew, as physicians, we wouldn't be allowed "outside the wire," meaning allowed off base. Physicians, especially surgeons, were in short supply, so it was a rare doctor who was allowed to travel around unencumbered like I did three years before. Hell, I doubted we'd even be allowed to dip a toe into the sand outside the fence.

As we lounged in our tent, I offered one piece of what I hoped was sage advice: don't talk politics. I had a feeling the group was fairly split when it came to conservative versus liberal, with me sitting smack dab on the center post of the political fence, but I knew the minute we started talking politics, we would implode as a group. We all agreed to put political opinions to pasture for the duration.

Weather in Iraq seemed to be a big issue—sandstorms were walloping the country, grounding a lot of aircraft, especially those transporting fresh troops into the war zone. After close to a week of false alarms, we got word we'd join a larger group on an eight o'clock evening flight to Tikrit. So, in a classic hurry-up-and-wait, we packed our duffels yet again and chain-carried them to the loading area at 2 P.M. The staging terminal was actually several miles from the airfield, and in some ways reminded me of an overcrowded Greyhound bus terminal. It was open-air, with separate roped-off areas under thin corrugated metal roofs that seemed to magnify rather than protect from the rays of the sun. Penned like cattle, we found scores of roasting soldiers lined up for the day's flights: Baghdad, Mosul, Taji, Q-West, and many more destinations; some names I recognized, others seemed completely foreign, which was appropriate considering they were foreign, at least to us tourists.

Our group sat until 5 P.M. behind the chalkboard that said "Tikrit" and were thankful when we were finally herded onto a bus that took us straight to the airfield and our C-130 sitting on the tarmac. We were told to drink as much as we could, use the porta-johns, then hold tight. The "hold tight" part lasted more than two hours as the plane sat and repetitively revved its engines. Finally, an Air Force guy walked over and gave us the bad news: no flight, engine problems. Sorry, fellas.

Bummed out, we filed onto the bus and headed back to the terminal. At the halfway point, the bus unexpectedly pulled a multi-g-force U-turn and zoomed back to the airfield. Problem solved, the flight was a now a hurry-up-and-go. We once again formed our weaving antlike procession, and funneled onto the plane through its rear ramp door.

On board we found we had more people than seats, but flying the friendly skies of the U.S. Air Force meant you never had to worry about being bumped—the human shoehorn technique worked for them. The inside of our C-130 was like any other, a dimly lit tube with two long parallel aisles, sort of like narrow hallways, where the web seats faced each other. It was a claustrophobe's nightmare: our knees touched the knees of the people across from us and we had to twist our shoulders at a weird angle so we'd all fit. The overbooking also meant your butt didn't exactly fit into the natural groove of the webbing; instead most of us were treated to metal support rods trying to give us a rectal exam through our uniforms. As the ramp of the plane closed, applause and whistles traveled up and down the line of seats. But the cheers dissolved into grumbles, then curses, as we continued to sit on the tarmac for another hour feeling the coarse vibrations of the engines being tested and retested by a sadistic pilot.

Problem solved my ass. If it was 120 degrees outside the plane, it had to be 30 degrees hotter inside. And we were in full battle rattle with Kevlar helmets, flak vests, and combat gear—to say nothing of the overstretched bladders from all the water we were told to drink. We wanted to document our suffering for some complaint-to-be-filed-later to the secretary of the air force, but the pictures we took didn't come out—it was so hot and humid in the flying oven, the lenses of our cameras fogged over. The sweat ran like a broken faucet from inside our helmets and poured off our chins. When a few of the guys started getting lethargic and began to heave, we knew heatstroke was imminent and this playing with the engines bullshit had to stop.

A young crewmember in a brown jumpsuit came back and said it would just be a few minutes more; his open mouth was met with the threat of a bullet to the head if the ramp wasn't opened—*now*. There was no way we were going to keel over from heat injury because of some asshole jerking around with the engines. It was shit or get off the plane. At first, I don't think he believed his passengers were serious, but we were already in group protection mode. None of us was going to sit quietly as one of our own collapsed from heatstroke. Wide-eyed, the airman watched as a hand reached toward a holster, only to be saved by a sudden jerk forward that told us we were either on our way to Tikrit . . . or the nearest jail.

The flight took less than an hour. Since C-130s aren't insulated, we shivered most of the trip as our sweat turned to ice water when we reached flying altitude. A few of the guys said the hell with it, and simply pissed their pants to relieve bladder spasms and abdominal pain. No bag of peanuts and a soft drink on this flight. Deliverance came with a landing that was different from any other I'd done before in the Army—rather than spiral in from ten thousand feet in a stomach-dropping free fall to avoid an enemy rocket, we skimmed the tree-tops at high speed for miles before the wheels kissed the pavement. Cramps were rubbed from muscles and wobbly knees gingerly tested before we filed off into the night and re-formed as a group. Once again, we stood and stared like lost children, wondering where we were and who would help us. The questions were answered quickly as a group of brand-new black Chevy Suburbans appeared from the darkness—it was a group from the hospital sent to fetch us and our belongings.

It seemed like we drove forever. The hospital was located within the confines of cavernous COB Speicher, with the COB standing for "Contingency Operating Base"—the military's new term for huge, monstrous, and probably-going-to-be-here-forever base. The COB was home of the 82nd Airborne's and 25th Infantry Division's main operations, with the 399th combat support hospital a flyspeck, but an important flyspeck, on its periphery. And as the former home of Saddam's Air Force Academy, there were a few concrete buildings left standing after the intense bombing raids of the war's first days. And we lucked out; one of those intact structures was to be our barracks. It wasn't much to look at. Pockmarked by bullet holes and shrapnel, the building was the same dull brown that seemed to be the color of paint the entire country was dipped in.

To our delight, we were handed new, unopened packages of sheets and pillowcases along with room assignments. To my further delight, I was bunking in what was called the "Love Shack," the largest room in the building, and the only one making up the third floor. By American standards, the "large" was relative—most of the other guys doubled up in plywood-sided rooms the size of a typical bathroom; mine was the size of three bathrooms. My roommates were my fellow ER doc Mike Barron and surgeon Ian Nunnally. As we walked through the door, our sleep-deprived brains blurrily did the math: three guys plus two beds equals a big problem. Our eyes twitched back and forth, and to each other—seeing who was going to blink first. Jarhead Mike solved the dilemma. Spying a homemade plywood table, Mike plopped his sleeping bag down and was snoring in less than a minute. He slept on that rickety platform every night for the next three months.

PARADISE GENERAL HOSPITAL

THE FEW HOURS of sleep I got that night were edgy—helicopters zipped through the night skies over Camp Speicher with an unpredictable regularity—each angry whirl of the blades kept me from fading into a much-needed sleep. I was disoriented but knew the hospital was close—and it seemed like every copter was making a drop-off outside my window. They must have had a busy night. All too soon, it would be my face waiting at the end of the line as the birds carried in their bloody cargo.

I pulled on my uniform and decided to make my way over to what would be my workplace for the next few months. Breakfast was out of the question—acid had eaten a hole in the lining of my stomach and I had a bad case of the jitters. As I opened the door on to the gravel-covered compound, the heat struck like a torch and the explosive rays of the desert sun took my vision away. *Jesus, don't forget to keep water with you all the time. And get some good sunglasses.* Several soldiers stared at me as I tentatively staggered across the blinding landscape. To them, I must have looked like a lost sheep searching for the rest of the flock. *Must be one of the new doctors,* their faces said.

I swallowed my embarrassment and decided to ask for directions.

"Morning, how's it going, guys?"

"Just fine, sir. Another day in fucking paradise."

"Can you tell me where the hospital is?"

"Just behind those walls, sir."

I mumbled a thanks and stared at the huge blast walls less than fifty yards away.

The short route was covered with gravel—in fact, the whole camp looked to be landscaped with the chunky gray rocks—and even at 7 A.M. the heat radiating off the gravel felt as if it were melting the rubber soles of my boots.

As I neared the hospital, another group of soldiers came by, snapping salutes as they passed.

"Morning, sir!"

I saluted back as I crunched along, "Hi, guys, how's it going?"

In unison, they answered, "Just another day in fucking paradise. Thank you, sir."

It was a phrase I would hear repeated several times more that morning, as well as every single morning for the rest of my deployment: "Another day in fucking paradise."

Bingo! We now had an official name for our new workplace: Paradise General Hospital.

I wasn't sure what to expect when I saw Paradise General for the first time. I knew it wasn't going to look like Johns Hopkins, but I wasn't ready for a group of shabby tents hidden behind the blast walls. It made the grounds of the 4077th MASH on TV seem like that of a major medical center. Out of the five combat support hospitals in Iraq, all had regular buildings and hard roofs except one. Ours. The bulk of our hospital was made up of a group of huge green tents with an occasional connection to an old building or to some trailers you'd typically see on the back of a semi, all surrounded by ten-foot-high, three-foot-thick blast walls to protect us from the rockets and mortars the insurgents would lob onto our laps. The support staff of more than two hundred had already been in country for a year and gone through three rotations of doctors—we were their fourth and final group—so they probably were elated to see us, even if they didn't know or trust us.

It was key I got off on the right foot at my new workplace; instead, I stepped in a verbal pothole and fell flat on my face. As I continued my openmouthed wandering, I realized another soldier was passing as I entered through a break in the blast walls. I spied a colonel's rank on the cap, which meant I needed to offer a salute and a greeting. Yet this superior officer had a few strands of long hair sticking out of the cap. Was this colonel a he or a she? It was like Vegas in Iraq, with 50–50 odds I'd guess the correct gender. I took a shot and bet on the hair.

"Morning, ma'am," I said with a confident air of respect and courtesy.

The stunned, pissed look told me I had rolled snake eyes.

A deep masculine voice replied, "Good . . . mor-ning . . . Ma-jor."

Shit!

He was one of the main bosses of the hospital. And it took less than ten seconds to get on his personal shit list thanks to my blurry-eyed gender confusion. I quickly mumbled an incoherent "Sir" and took off, stumbling past a collection of dusty tents. I had just had my initial encounter with an "administrator"—which in this camp was a four-letter word, especially one small group in particular, whose specialty was manufacturing misery for the medical staff.

The sign on the door of the ER said, "STOP! AUTHORIZED PERSONNEL ONLY!" in oversized block letters. Was I now authorized? Or did I have to wait until I went through my orientation and became official before entering the no-man's-land of the emergency room? I took a deep breath, rolled the dice again, and pushed through the doors. It was like stepping from a serene forest into a multicar pileup. Blood, screaming, and a kaleidoscope of chaos.

"Can I help you, sir?"

Help me?

"Ah, well, I'm one of the new docs."

"Welcome, sir, we heard you folks got in last night. Get you a cup of coffee?"

I snuck a peek at the sergeant's nametag—"Courage." He was the NCOIC of the ER—the noncommissioned officer in charge. And I could use a dose of his name right now. He sat calmly at a desk despite the yelling and screaming that peeled the paint off the walls. A bloody stump of an arm hung off one stretcher, while on the next one over a Niagara of blood poured onto the floor as a group of medics struggled to cinch tight a tourniquet around where a leg used to be. The other leg pointed oddly at a right angle away from the body at the knee.

"Sure, coffee would be great—a beer would be better."

In a thick New England accent he said, "I know what you mean, sir, but all we've got is the black gasoline—and come to think of it, foo-foo at that."

Foo-foo?

I filled an empty cup and wandered down the line of stretchers toward the action—watching as IV lines were stuck blindly into the deep veins of the neck and groin and morphine injected to quiet the screams of men whose bodies had been assaulted by shrapnel. Blood flowed on the floor in a small stream, collecting in grooves and cracks of the crusty linoleum. Fresh blood has a unique smell—tangy with a bitter sweetness—and this morning it penetrated and attached itself to the deepest lining of my nose. I sipped at the coffee, hoping to wash away the putrid fragrance, and wound up spitting out a small mouthful in surprise. It was Almond Spice—one of the many flavors of "foo-foo" coffees favored by a crew who struggled for some sense of sensual calm in the face of daily carnage. I staggered out of the overcrowded room, fighting the rising bile in the back of my throat as I realized in a few days I'd be on the game field, not watching from the bleachers.

Before we were allowed any hands-on work, we all had to go through orientation—starting with a day-long PowerPoint presentation and a series of briefings on the rules of the camp, rules of the hospital, lab procedures, blood protocols, schedule of religious services, all piled onto an overflowing plate of topics no one paid attention to or remembered. But one thing did stand out: it seemed almost every female who gave a lecture spent a lot of time staring at the well-built body of the gently snoring Bernard Harrison as they spoke.

The briefings were held in a musty dark gray tent with a reluctant air conditioner, which combined with bewildered body clocks left us looking like a bunch of bobblehead dolls, lolling off to sleep, then jerking back to consciousness. Tumbling in late came Billy Stanton, who won the prize for the first to get onto the playing field. Last night, the copters I heard were ferrying wounded, and Bill never went to bed; staying up and helping the soon-to-depart overworked orthopedist with a series of amputations, compound fractures, and limbs torn to shreds by the hot fragments of roadside bombs.

"Holy shit, dude, it was some nasty stuff."

He and the other surgeon had only just finished the cases I had wandered into that morning in the ER. In a place where almost everyone who came through the door had something blown off, torn off, or broken off, there was one orthopedist when there should have been four. Soon it would be Bill who was operating night and day without help.

Next up was a quick meet with the medical boss, Dr. Greg Quick, the kindly colonel who had picked us up at the airfield the night before. Greg was an ER doc from Massachusetts who opted to spend an entire year with the 399th supervising the groups of doctors rotating through the facility. Just around the corner from the mandatory retirement of age sixty, Greg wore oversized glasses that spotlighted his quirky facial expressions, which mainly consisted of a bemused ability to raise his gray eyebrows all the way to his hairline while talking. His voice was high-pitched and he had a consistent way of finishing a statement with a rising question mark of "Hmm?" We had no clue of how bad his year had been to this point but would gradually learn how far he would go out of his way to make sure "his doctors" were taken care of, as well as keeping us one step ahead of the Army's "stupid rule" police.

"Your only job is to take care of patients—that's pretty simple, wouldn't you say, hmm?"

He filled us in on some of the unpleasantries of our stay: we were short a surgeon and two ER docs, so we'd be pulling extra shifts. Greg's voice was soft and cheery, as if discussing a gorgeous springtime morning instead of one with ominous clouds and deadly tornadoes in the forecast.

Sure, Mike and Dave, we know you're family doctors but since you each have ER experience in the States, we're all sure you can handle trauma here—but we'll talk about that later in private. And Dave, we know you can work a scalpel so maybe you could help out the surgeons when you're not in the ER. And don't worry, you'll all have some free time—but not really—you're technically on twenty-four-hour-a-day call every day of the deployment. Sorry, we have no phones to the barracks—we use pagers to communicate with the doctors. Going anywhere, including the latrine, without your pager is a sin punishable by screaming. We wouldn't want that, would we, hmmm? Oh, one more, sorry, but you do have to salute outside the hospital compound—but inside we are a no-salute zone. And don't forget to take your cap off when you enter the hospital grounds, we wouldn't want something sucked into the engine of a medevac, hmmm? Finally, we don't do neurological or facial surgery here—the one phone we do have has a direct connection to the Air Force hospital in Balad. They've got specialists—use them.

We sat there stunned trying to soak in all in.

A few minutes later, we broke for lunch and a self-conducted mini-tour of the camp. The blast furnace outside was actually a relief from the musty steam of the overcrowded tent. As we pushed through the flap, Bernard said, "I've got a feeling we are in for a fucking hell of a ride." Grim nods all around.

Few words were spoken as we crunched our way toward the DFAC or dining facility. We'd seen a glimpse of it last night when we arrived, but in daylight were surprised at its mammoth size: easily two football fields with seating for a few thousand. Quite a difference from the little fifty-person fly-infested shitholes that fed me during my first tour. The shiny concrete and steel DFAC was newly built and quite a contrast to our hospital of drab tents. After armed guards checked our IDs, we were directed to a mandatory hand-washing station, then finally into the DFAC itself. Stationed at the door was an enlisted soldier whose sole job was to work the "clicker," a little handheld counter than clicked every time a diner entered the facility. And each click was $32 into the pocket of some faceless multigazillion-dollar civilian corporation. Not a bad business deal, figuring the Camp Speicher megacomplex fed more than fourteen thousand soldiers and contractors three meals a day. Do the math and it totaled a nice *1.3 million dollars a day*—give or take a few hundred thousand bucks for skipped meals. Not that the service, at first glance, didn't seem worth it—we were waited on by bow-tied white-shirted contract workers from countries such as Sri Lanka and Indonesia. But the food choices left a little to be desired. The menu moved through a three-week cycle of deep-fried, artery-clogging monotony. If something could be cooked in a deep fryer, in it went, except for fresh-off-the-grill burgers, which we suspected were actually ground camel; mushy fruit that had suffered through countless cycles of freezing and thawing on its journey to us; and honest-to-goodness stir-fry, though we were never sure exactly *what* was being stirred and fried.

On the plus side were huge refrigerators filled with soda, Gatorade, and chocolate milk, which sat on the periphery of the huge hall, right next to the plasma flat screens that typically showed sports or political programming. I grabbed what looked like a Diet Pepsi from the fridge, but a closer look revealed its foreign lettering. I think Turkish, which proclaimed "Harika Tat!" in big letters. The translation, we later learned, was "Tastes Great!" I watched Rick stuff six cans into his now bulging cargo pockets—while I was the coffee addict, his vice was consuming gallons of diet soda each day.

We sat munching our fare at long tables with clean plastic-covered white tablecloths that were meticulously brushed of crumbs when our meals were finished. Lest you leave your sweet tooth unsatisfied, you could top off your meal with an assortment of cakes, pies, brownies, and ten different flavors of ice cream—they'd even make you a sundae if you asked. Maybe that's what the $32 was spent on, because it sure wasn't health food. The battle of Iraq for many rear-echelon and support troops was really the battle of the bulge—the average weight gain of a soldier serving a year in Iraq was 10.5 pounds. This was definitely not my father's war with its K rations, nor my 2004 tour with MREs or little cans of ravioli.

We had about ten minutes to make it back to our orientation—and that was about nine more than we needed. COB Speicher was a huge base, about twenty square miles in size—little wonder it took so long to get from the airfield to our barracks the night before. With the pounding the base had taken in the early days of the war, craters dotted the landscape. As it was slowly transformed into an American superbase, the camp now had paved roads, bus lines, and stop signs—as well as military police with radar guns who would issue a ticket to the poor Humvee driver who exceeded the 10 mph speed limit.

Yet most of us would never see that part of the world; we were cautioned not to venture off the miniature half-mile-square section tucked into a distant corner of the base. Our little universe consisted of barracks, DFAC, hospital, gym, shower trailers, and latrines, so closely nestled, all could be reached in three minutes—and in the case of an emergency run to the latrine, fifty-two seconds. All routes were covered by those ankle-twisting chunks of hot gravel. We wondered how long it took them to truck it all in and where in heaven they got it from. The distance from the DFAC to the hospital was literally a gravel throw.

As we reentered the orientation sauna tent, we were sentenced to more Death by PowerPoint—but this time we walked through slides overflowing with information we actually needed to learn: resuscitation guidelines, head trauma and blunt abdominal trauma protocols, transfer procedures, hypothermia and shock, use of whole blood and some experimental blood-clotting product with a science-fiction-type name: recombinant factor VIIa. I was blown away and panicked at being force-fed an avalanche of material—then having to know it inside and out within the next twenty-four hours. The others seemed to squirm in their seats as well. Rick gently elbowed me and whispered a reassuring, "We'll be okay." He was right: if we each learned the basics, then picked one topic to become expert on, we could bail each other out. But I still felt like I was now in a brave new world, and I was feeling more and more like a coward. *God, please don't let me hurt anyone.*

In walked Colonel Brent Smith, the current head of emergency services, who was slated to leave in a couple of days. Although he was supposedly years younger than most of us, he shuffled slowly and had deep crevices around his eyes that surrounded thick bags of fatigue. His tour had been rough, and a three-month collection of trauma cases deeply etched his face. Smith was loved by the staff and had a stellar reputation as a trauma doc. He spoke in a near whisper.

"Hi, everybody. I need you all to hook up with your counterparts for right seat/left seat this afternoon."

Right seat/left seat was the Army policy similar to a pilot/copilot situation on an airplane. We would be the copilots until we learned how the CSH flew, then we would move into the left seat and be in charge. The normal right seat/left seat orientation takes five to seven days. We would have one with maybe a second if lucky.

Brent gave what sounded like a canned spiel about the hospital, and then told everyone to get lost except for the three ER trauma docs. Gerry, Mike, and I sat quietly as Brent explained the cases we would be seeing, and how most of the wounds would challenge even the most experienced trauma surgeon. As family practitioners, Mike and I were terrific at treating colds or giving flu shots, and while Gerry was an actual ER doc he never saw IEDs in Cleveland. There was no question we would be like first-day interns who were suddenly told to perform brain surgery. Colonel Quick sat quietly in the corner of the tent as he waited for Brent to finish scaring the shit out of us. He could clearly read the anxiety on our faces and after giving us a few seconds to let things sink in, told us we could accept our assignments in the ER, or instead, take a more comfortable job staffing the sick call clinic. No questions or loss of respect, the hospital would get by. One by one, we answered. Gerry: yes. Mike: yes. Me: Uh, I'm scared shitless. Quick: That's the best answer I've heard yet. You'll do fine. Across the tent, Brent's sad eyes sagely nodded agreement.

I didn't sleep well that night, or, for that matter, any night for the next few months. The helicopters returned en masse with their overnight deliveries and I tossed and turned as each one whizzed by our barracks. By now, I had a little better sense of direction—I realized if I simply looked out the window of our rooftop room to the southeast, I could peer over the blast walls and make out the blue landing lights of the helipad at the hospital. It hit me: many of the birds zooming by were actually Cobra attack helicopters or Black Hawks ferrying troops on and off the base, not incoming medevacs. I only saw a few of the speeding shadows make use of the vaguely lit landing zone of Paradise General. But even a few meant the doctors who we would replace within the next twenty-four hours were getting hammered.

THE NEXT MORNING started with three large cups of weak coffee and a bowl of Cheerios drowning in semiwarm milk poured from a carton with Turkish lettering. Ka-chingg! For $32, I could have had a gourmet breakfast with seconds and thirds back in the States.

The medical menu for the day showed us breaking into small groups and following our counterparts to finish our right seat/left seat orientation. Gerry, Mike, and I tracked down Brent Smith as he helped another doc clear the ER of a group of soldiers jolted around by an IED. Except for a couple of bloody eardrums, the men looked stunned yet relatively unscathed. *Doesn't look too bad*, I thought. *Maybe I can do this.*

We attacked the computer system first. Everything was documented in a very standard and regimented format, and it was important that we got this part right. The medical records would follow wounded soldiers to places like Landstuhl Medical Center in Germany, Walter Reed in D.C., and the burn center at Brooke Army Medical Center in San Antonio.

"Try to make sure you're accurate. Other docs will be reading what the original injuries were and what you did to fix them." Brent rapped the desk with his fist for emphasis as he talked.

"And it's especially important for disability and brain injuries that everything gets documented—some of the subtle things don't show up for months after a guy goes home and you don't want him to get screwed out of benefits and care, especially if he's in the National Guard or Reserves."

His fingers flew across the keyboard as he wrapped up a complete record in less than two minutes.

"It'll take you twenty minutes to get it right the first few times. Don't worry about it—do a few hundred and you'll be able to knock a medical record out in thirty seconds while taking care of a bunch of bleeders at the same time. Remember how the old Army ran on paper? The new one runs on electrons—all computers. And by the way, forget all that new computer shit they taught you in Kuwait, this is a different system."

We then took a quick tour of the ER itself. Although the majority of the hospital was made up of tents and containers, the ER was one of the few structures that actually had a hardened roof—"the best place to be if you get mortared." The ER was long and narrow, with a door at each end. It had six trauma "bays"—lettered "A" (Alpha) through "F" (Foxtrot). Alpha was furthest from the front door and was reserved for the most severe cases since it was only steps to the OR tent and intensive care unit through the rear door. Over the next few months, I would find myself standing in Alpha straining my neck watching stretchers with the critically wounded traversing the thirty-five feet from front door to me—sometimes they seemed to come too fast, before I felt ready, other times agonizingly slow as life's blood dripped onto the floor.

Brent handed us papers with diagrams like football plays—the most important showed our positioning during a trauma case. Most of the bays contained no stretchers—we would use what the patient came in on—and we physicians would pre-position ourselves at the upper-right-hand side of the bay where the stretcher would be parked headfirst. Next to us at the head of the patient would be a respiratory tech or an anesthetist. In various positions around the stretcher would be a medic to insert a right-side IV, another medic for a left-side IV, a circulating medic, a medication nurse, an X-ray tech, and a recording nurse, who wrote down any medication or blood administered. Everyone had a position to play and a job to do.

"Then there's the red line." Brent punched out the words as if they were the most important he would ever say.

We looked at a long red painted line a few feet away from the foot of where the stretcher would be.

"No one crosses that line unless you say so. Surgeons and gas passers love to jump in and get their hands dirty right away—don't let them. Everyone stays behind the line until you do your assessment, get your lines in, and start treatment. Otherwise, it's like dinner for twenty in a small phone booth. If you don't hear one other thing today, hear this: you are the boss in this room—get pushed around and someone will die."

His words made me shiver. I'd never done this stuff before and now I was supposed to be ordering smarter people around while some kid is gurgling blood.

With relief, we left the ER through the far door and saw that fifteen steps away after a sharp left turn was the OR. At least we were told it was the OR. All I saw was a blanket covering the opening of a tent.

Smith saw our openmouthed stares.

"It's nothing fancy, but a lot of lives get saved in there. Two tables. Three in a pinch. Plus it's a close ride on a stretcher."

We looked down and saw droplets of blood mark the journey from the ER to the OR blanket. A couple of dots, then a streak, followed by a series of thick beads of congealed red globs. I wanted, yet didn't want, to know what waited behind that mysterious woolen blanket.

We took a quick right and walked to a long cavernous tent—the PLX: Pharmacy/Lab/X-ray. Nothing special until we saw the ultra-modern CAT scanner, which was very cool to have—until we realized what we didn't have to go with it: a radiologist. Back home CAT scans were a godsend, and so were the people who could interpret them. Need an image of a brain? I would ask the nurse to order a CAT scan, the test would be done, and then I'd get a report within minutes from the radiologist telling me what the CAT showed. Instant gratification. Now I had a problem of monumental proportion. I had interpreted exactly *zero* CAT scans in my career, and now I would be on the firing line in the middle of the night, by myself, trying to determine if that little black spot was a simple shadow or bleeding in the brain. I'd give up my firstborn for a radiologist.

Just then, the tent started shaking as a pair of helicopters skidded in for a quick landing. No warning. We hustled back to the ER in time to see a couple of stretchers come in, blood-streaked arms hanging over the sides as the wheels spun toward Alpha and Bravo bays. Just like the playbook, everyone was in position and ready to work. The activity seemed like a blender—lots of buzzing noise and lots of swirling activity, none of which seemed to make sense. From behind the red line, all I could see was burnt strips of flesh hanging off a pair of legs, bright white shards of bone sticking through bloody holes of clothing, and the constant drip-drip of blood onto the floor from a saturated dressing wrapped around a wound in the arm. I stuffed my hands into my pockets so no one would notice the shaking. It would be this group's last trauma cases of their deployment—at midnight they would hand the baton to us. On quaking legs, I walked back to my room when the cases were finished, tried reading a borrowed copy of *CAT Scans for Dummies*, and then asked God what I had done to piss him off.

FIRST DAY OF SCHOOL

THE HELICOPTER BLADES chopped through the night air, and once again chopped through my sleep. I had maybe one solid forty-five-minute stretch of undisturbed slumber, but even that was infiltrated by a bad dream.

Through all of my years of schooling and training, I'd had a lot of first days—this one was by far the worst. For every step I took toward the hospital, I wanted to take two steps back. Inhaling a breath of bravery, I pushed open the door to the ER, and must have had a "deer in the headlights" look as I peered in.

"No, you're not lost. Glad you decided to come to work today, sir."

It was my friendly coffee NCO, Sergeant Courage.

"I bet you could go for a nice hot cup of coffee, huh, sir? None of that foo-foo shit today—we just got in a shipment from home of Dunkin' Donuts high-test."

"Thank God. That stuff yesterday was like water from the bottom of a flower vase. What kind of coffee surprises do you guys hide in here?" I asked.

"Pumpkin Spice, Cinnamon Tulip, French Butternut, and all that kind of horseshit." He swiveled his head toward the staff. "They like it but give me a cup of regular java anyday. Nothing like liquid artillery to welcome the morning."

The place looked like a foreign land, and as I scanned the room, I was surprised at how young the medics were. Some of them looked like they had just been introduced to a razor. With an average age of maybe twenty-three, they had already seen enough carnage to last several lifetimes. Many had no background in medicine before being deployed; some were carpenters, some were schoolteachers, and others full-time college students. All were reservists and all had volunteered to spend fifteen months of their lives saving lives. And they were very good at it. The hospital boasted a survival rate of more than 95 percent, which meant we new docs were under some serious pressure to perform. They silently stared and tightly nodded greetings as Courage handed me my full cup of high-octane. As I nodded back, I could read their thoughts: *Is this guy stupid or smart, arrogant or cool? And what about the rest of the doctors? Just who and what were they?* It wouldn't be until the first trauma case that we'd *all* truly find out.

I wandered the narrow room, shaking hands with each of the medics lounging in folding chairs—they were all young enough to be my children.

"Hi, I'm Major Hnida but you can call me Dave."

"Yes, sir, glad to meet you."

"Welcome to our little corner of the universe, Dr. Hnida."

"Hello, Major, how are you?"

So much for informalities. I didn't do well with the "Major" label, was uncomfortable with the "Sir" business, and the only one who called me "Doctor" was my overly proud mother. I'd have to work on this name stuff.

Next up were staff nurses—all worked in emergency rooms back home and probably had more knowledge of trauma medicine in their pinkies than I knew altogether. Just like home, I knew a doctor's best allies were the nurses. All you had to do was listen and they'd guide you safely down unknown paths.

Last to be introduced were the head nurses in charge of the department. Both held the rank of major. Roger Boutin was a firefighter and nurse from rural Massachusetts. With thick-rimmed glasses and a high and tight crew cut, Roger looked like a rigid throwback to the Army of the Cold War—but I would learn he had a love of the classics, the eclectics such as Jack Kerouac, and was responsible for the bottomless supply of foo-foo coffee that kept everyone mellow.

Boutin was the assistant to Jack Twomey, a stoic figure whose imposing demeanor told me his ER ship was a tight one. Twomey was an ER nurse in one of Boston's busiest trauma centers and probably could staff this department all by himself—no doctors needed, or for that matter, even wanted. It would take weeks for me to learn the motives behind Twomey's firm expectations—for now, I worried he would eat me for lunch, then spit the bones out after picking his teeth.

As the introductions finished, Sergeant Courage tapped me on the elbow.

"One firm rule in the ER, sir, all weapons go into the lockbox at the front desk. We'll show you where we hide the key."

That made sense. In the confusion of a busy emergency room you didn't want any weapons within reach of a insurgent, or for that matter a pissed-off soldier who has just seen his buddy blown up. I foggily recalled part of a briefing during orientation the day before. Not only was everyone disarmed in the ER, every patient brought in was relieved of their firearms and grenades, and in the case of an Iraqi—insurgent or otherwise—strip-searched for weapons and things like suicide vests before leaving the helipad. Sometimes the enemy was obvious, but a few of the bad guys hid in the uniforms of Iraqi police or army and caution was the word of this war. I reached down, unstrapped my pistol, and locked it away. It was a place I would learn to lock my emotions as well.

I set my stethoscope down and got the nickel tour of the ER from Courage. Although I had been here before, now the view was different, like seeing it from the playing field instead of the grandstands. I had combat patches on my uniform from my first deployment that caught some attention as we strolled down the narrow row of six trauma bays. But to hell with the patches: if I didn't perform well in those trauma bays, this crew wouldn't want me soiling their turf.

I then went through each bay and opened drawers, studied equipment hanging on walls, and tried to get a sense of the trauma gear that bulged out of every nook and cranny. One of the medics stopped me as I finished my inventory.

"You're the first doctor I've ever seen do that, you know, check out the gear. That's good, sir, you must know what you're doing. We've had a couple of real losers come through here. Don't get me wrong, almost all of them were great docs but one or two fucking sucked. Made our lives hell." A heartbeat of a pause. "Sir."

I murmured a weak thanks and wondered how I'd be judged when our last day came in a September I couldn't even see on the horizon. I wondered if any of them could see through my veneer of confidence. If they only knew how scared I was, how poorly equipped I felt to do this job, how I wondered how I got myself into this mess. If they only knew.

We didn't get a lot of time to socialize before my first case came limping through the door. It was a soldier who sprained his ankle playing basketball at the camp gym. My head spun for a second: I came to Iraq for this? This is the same crap I see at home. The medics did a mini-exam and ordered an X-ray.

"Looks negative to me, sir, I think we can just give him some ranger candy and send him out."

"Ranger candy?"

"Ibuprofen, sir. They gobble it like M&Ms."

I doubled-checked the ankle and the X-ray and agreed.

Patient number two was a young soldier with "desert cough" that was keeping him awake all night. Once again, a mini-exam and a trip over for a chest X-ray. So far, I had been in the clinic for almost an hour and had done little except sit and watch everyone else care for patients.

It took only five more minutes before I got to taste the first appetizer of what my next few months would serve on a bloody platter. I was just resigning myself to the painful task of looking at the medical records system on the computer when the metal doors swung inward with a bang. I looked up to see a group of American soldiers half dragging in a moaning Iraqi soldier with bloody ears that were hanging by thin threads of skin. Insurgents had been slowly slicing the ears off in the back room of a small house when a group of American troops burst in to save the day.

In the States, the Iraqi would have been sent to a specialist. Here he came to me. Not only were the ears barely attached, but what was left hanging had been sliced and diced with a sharp blade. The cuts looked like the roadmap to hell and the strips of skin looked like they would flutter in a stiff breeze. I stared at the ears, not knowing what part was supposed to go where. The main pieces were still bleeding so I knew I still had some vessels attached—now all I needed to do was quilt the bloody puzzle back together. I tried to hide my panic from the staff and set out to work, praying the doctor fairy would miraculously come through the door with an Ear, Nose, and Throat specialist.

As I cross-stitched and knitted away, word came over the radio of my first American trauma case. A soldier shot through the neck by a sniper. The estimated arrival time was twenty minutes. But I couldn't hear the rest of the details. The loud rotor blades of a landing chopper and the pounding of running feet drowned out all conversation. Show time . . . and I hadn't been to rehearsal. I looked up to see Greg Quick walk through the door.

"Sounds like you've got business, hmm?" He shot a quick glance at the ears. "This will take me five minutes, you take care of the important stuff."

Five minutes to fix the ears? Important stuff? American shot through the neck? I thought they said twenty minutes. I was drowning in confusion.

I scrambled to Alpha bay and took my place at the head, where the stretcher would roll to a stop. As I slipped on gloves and work goggles, I saw our little ER quickly fill up. News travels quickly when an American is coming in by chopper and every doctor, clerk, administrator, and staff member hustled in for a front-seat view of the action. Even the doctors we relieved came over from their quarters—their plane wasn't due to leave until tonight. Plus, I realized Quick didn't come over to help me mend some ears—he'd come to watch my performance.

There was a flurry of movement throughout the room and an eruption of noise as the stretcher burst through the door. *Holy shit.* It was a skinny young kid with a sickly gray cast to his skin. A leg jaggedly pointed at an unnatural angle; actually, what was left of the leg. And a thick bandage around his neck saturated with blood. It had to be a carotid or a jugular wound. As the stretcher moved into the bay, medics quickly scrambled to place IV lines while I stared at the tiny bubbles forming on the surface of the bandage. Each bubble grew large, then small with the rhythmic chest compressions of CPR.

In my mind, the room went pitch black, with a single, bright spotlight focused on me, and me alone. In the middle of a vast stage, every eye in the audience was now focused on me and awaiting my impersonation of a qualified trauma leader. It should have been about the guy on the stretcher, but no, in my mind, it was all about me and whether I was up to the task of being allowed to perform on the Broadway of the emergency room.

I simply didn't know where to start—or maybe I did know, but couldn't. I just stood there, staring. In the meantime, Major Twomey was at the foot of the stretcher, waiting for me to begin my assessment of the patient—describing, in order, status of the airway, the soldier's breathing, his circulation, and level of consciousness. It was all cookbook medicine but I couldn't remember a word of the recipe.

I could faintly hear Twomey's voice, but it was like a distant echo, muffled as if we were underwater. There was a racing beep from the heart monitor but I couldn't tell if it was the patient's heart hammering away, or my own. Numbers were being shouted out—they could have been blood pressure readings or medication orders, I couldn't tell. And yelling from the peanut gallery—*Don't touch that dressing! Get some pressure on that wound! Take off that dressing, you've got to see where that bleeding is coming from! He needs an airway! Call for blood! Let X-ray get in there!*

Then came a sudden parting of the sea as a mass of doctors rushed toward and then swarmed around the patient—each with their own idea of what needed to be done. Alone in a crowded war, I was literally being pushed away from the head of the stretcher as the bodies crowded into the bay. There were no familiar faces for support or guidance, our new group was relegated to the periphery as the soon-to-depart doctors ordered the medics to wheel the patient straight to surgery. Rick, Bernard, and Ian followed at a distance.

As the stretcher flew out the door, the medics started swabbing blood from the floor, and Quick went back to mending his ears. All so routine. It was as if nothing serious had happened. As I stood trying to absorb what had just turned my world on its head, I felt someone roughly grab my arm. It was one of the hospital administrators, the "he" I had called a "she" the day I arrived on the base. He yanked me toward the door. "Get out there and talk to his unit. Tell them what's going on. It's your job to keep them informed. Now do it!"

About ten members of the soldier's unit had gathered just outside the ER, smoking, pacing, and anxiously talking among themselves. The gathering wasn't unusual; combat units were like a big family, and one soldier's wound made them all bleed.

Talking to family members and loved ones was a task I usually did well, but not today. I stumbled and fumbled over words that spilled out in a collection of confusion: *It looks like he's shot in the neck and the bullet hit a big blood vessel. The leg is bad, too. He's in surgery now. I don't know how long it's going to take, it's touch-and-go right now. I'm sorry but I wish I could tell you more. I just don't know.* So much for the reassuring manner of an experienced physician. I was an embarrassment.

I stepped away from the flapping blanket of the OR entrance and found a quiet spot between a couple of tents. I was so new I didn't know where I was, but my stomach didn't care. First, I threw up my coffee from breakfast, then some green bile, followed by a series of retches so violent there were spots of blood mixed in with the mucus. It took a few minutes for the dry heaves to slow and I weakly wiped the putrid residue off my uniform. *I can't do this shit. I'm going to hurt somebody.*

I had two choices—walk away claiming some bogus illness or do an about-face and face the music of my medical peers. The answer came in the form of a question: what would I tell my kids to do?

I spun around back into the ER and went straight to Major Twomey.

Can we speak outside?

He nodded and led the way to the helipad. We stopped on the first landing pad where I stared at my bloodied boots.

"I fucked up. Big-time."

"Well, it wasn't the most organized effort, but no, you didn't."

"I know a fuckup. And that was one. I got stampeded."

"Listen, you wouldn't be here if you couldn't do the job."

"Then level with me, what can I do better?"

"Easy. Be in charge. When we get a case, it's you, the medics, and me or Boutin. No one else in that room counts. No one. Don't let anyone cross that red line until you're ready for them. It was like a circus in there for a bit. You don't need twenty docs crowding you out of the way."

"Man, I screwed the pooch on this one."

"Just stop for a minute and look at one thing. We've got a guy who should be dead, but he's not. So you didn't make any fatal errors. Just go over your protocols until you can do them in your sleep. And be the boss. It's your ER when you are at the head of the stretcher."

"Thanks. And sorry."

"There's nothing to be sorry about. That's why it's called the practice of medicine. And at least you give a shit."

With that, Twomey abruptly spun on his heels and headed back to the ER.

Next on my list was Sergeant Courage.

Can we talk for a minute?

"Sir, whatever you need."

"I need your critique. That was a disaster in there. I fucked up."

"Well, I don't think you fucked up, sir, and I don't think any other people think you fucked up."

"I lost control."

"Sir, if you did, we couldn't tell. You looked nice and calm until the thundering herd of surgeons came into the bay. And they shouldn't have come in."

"My brain froze."

"Well, sir, we've got a live soldier in surgery right now. So it wasn't too frozen where you did something wrong. You'll be fine, sir. Just keep the place calm. We like calm."

"Thanks. I owe you one. And the medics, too."

"You don't owe us nothing, sir. Let's go have a cup of thunder, unless there's anything else, sir."

"No . . . nothing you can fix."

We walked back in through the swinging door and I scanned the room. Looking to see if any of the staff had dirty looks aimed in my direction. Nothing. They just went about their duties as if nothing had happened or, for that matter, had gone wrong. My shift had another eight hours to go and I prayed no more helicopters would be making deliveries.

I asked Twomey to pull the patient flow chart, which tracked the minute-by-minute happenings of the case. The sterile papers didn't reflect the chaos that took place in that room or in my head. I saw Twomey had filled in his sections . . . and mine as well. It all looked organized and clean. He had done a nice job covering my confusion. I sat squeezing the pain and the memories of the case from my forehead.

About an hour later, Rick and Bernard came out of the OR where they had watched the outgoing surgeons perform their final case.

"Looks like he's going to make it, man," Bernard said.

"Tough wound, though, transected the whole jugular right in half. Nicked a bunch of other stuff, too," Rick added. "I'm kind of amazed he didn't die on the spot. The other surgeons did a good job. He'll be in Germany by tonight."

Bernard looked at me oddly. "What's up with you, man? You look like shit."

"I feel like shit and I did my job like shit. I didn't exactly know what I was doing. It was like a zoo in here."

"Good lord mother of mercy. How many shot-in-the-jugulars have you ever seen? You must have one crazy-assed practice back home if you've seen any."

Rick now was staring, too.

"Dave, you look like this ole pregnant mare I had back on my farm. Did you eat anything today? Or you got morning sickness?"

"Not hungry. And I've got all-day sickness."

Bernard said, "C'mon, ease up on yourself, man. You did fine. Tell you what, hold down Fort Crazy here, and we'll see you in a bit."

My two lifelines strode from the room, whispering between themselves, leaving me to think, *I can't be trusted to be left alone in here. I know it, they know it, and the wounded probably know it.* As soon as the door swung shut, my heart jumped into my throat as I sensed, then felt, the rumbling vibration of a helicopter on approach. *Oh God.* I saw that the medics were already on their way out the door—*Jeez, they had no clue anything was coming*—I grabbed my stethoscope off the desk and began to pace. When eternity passed and the door swung back open, my eyes were pulled straight to the smile on the face of one of the medics.

"Just a blood run from Baghdad, sir. No business for us."

It was simply a helicopter replenishing our blood supply. I weakly smiled back, then went outside and threw up again.

By the time I cleaned myself up, Bernard and Rick were back waiting at my desk.

"The medical literature well documents a growing boy has got to eat. And you . . . are that growing boy," Bernard said with a hint of a smile.

Rick added, "Yeah, you gotta eat more than that royal shitburger you just got shoved down your throat."

On top of the desk was a buffet line of sandwiches, burgers, spaghetti, cake, even a puddle of chocolate ice cream that didn't survive the trip from the chow hall. My two friends tried to look tough and force me to take in some nourishment.

As they watched my mouth struggle to force down even the smallest bites, Rick said, "Now don't start thinking we did this because we like you. But if you die, then we all have to pick up extra shifts. And that ain't going to happen." It was a contest where make-believe glares lost out to grown-men giggles.

I was grateful for the gesture of nourishment and later realized it was the start of a ritual that lasted the next three months. I had lunch hand-delivered every day I worked an ER shift. And always made sure the surgeons had nourishment when they worked through mealtime.

I stayed until seven that night, and saw eight more patients. None were blown into pieces or had been shot; most had simple wounds or problems I could easily handle. I had survived day one, as did the shredded ears and the torn jugular. But there was no way I wanted to go back to work the next day; I almost wished for some near fatal disease to suddenly strike, the million-dollar illness—and with it, a ticket home. But that would be letting my friends down. My family down. Myself down.

HOT TAMALE

IT WAS ONE of those times I really missed having a dad. Someone to talk to, get advice from, maybe even to deliver a well-intentioned slap to the side of the head. I thought back to my terrifying night in the ditch back in '04; tonight I was in my ditch of 2007, crawling around feeling trapped and surrounded by fear.

I knew I couldn't leave. The fork in the road was well defined and I needed to choose the path of honor and decency, but I didn't know if I had the courage and the guts.

I pulled out my dad's wallet, and with it, a couple of pictures I hung under the top railing of my bunk. The first was a picture of a happy and innocent twenty-three-year-old in uniform sporting a wide grin. It was taken the day before he shipped out. Next to it, I hung the picture of him the day he came back—bandage on the forehead, dark circles surrounding hollow eyes, and a look that no words existed to describe. I stared at the pictures, begging for advice, some guidance, or words of encouragement. I wanted the easy answers, but they didn't come. Instead, I kept hearing what I didn't want to hear: Dave, choose the tough path—honor and decency.

What about my penance? I felt a duty to those I had failed in the past—the kids of Columbine, my daughter Katie, my own family, and the memory of my father. And the last now carried an extra burden. In reading my father's notes from his wallet and logbook, I had come across some scribbling on the tops, sides, and margins of several pages. By themselves, they made no sense; together they painted a clear picture of the pain he felt and the debt he believed he owed. A debt he briefly referred to during our long car ride to Philly, but gave little detail about as he quickly changed the subject. Now I understood, and here I had the chance to do what he couldn't. I could pay his sixty-year debt if I swallowed my fears and did my job.

I walked over to my footlocker and ripped open a packet of index cards. On each, I drew a series of flow charts for every conceivable situation that might show up in my ER. I knew I couldn't get them all, and I knew I probably wouldn't even have time to fumble through a big stack and pull out the right one when the shit hit the fan—but I would carry those cards with me at all times like a heart patient carries nitroglycerin to put under the tongue for sudden chest pain.

Before they went into the pocket of the uniform I'd wear tomorrow, I recited the protocols again and again—like a schoolchild repeating the newly learned alphabet—making sure I knew, by rote, the steps I would take, and the orders I would give when something came through the door. Even if I didn't do everything perfectly, I would at least do something—there would be no freezing, no chaos, in my ER ever again. I thought back to what my dad had told me about the first night he led a group of men on a patrol.

"It was pitch black and we walked right smack into a German ambush. Lots of gunfire, guys hit, screaming for medics. I wanted to burrow into the ground and stay there forever. Then my gut kicked in. You know, all those nights training and studying paid off. It's like memorizing your A-B-Cs."

It was 4 A.M. when I finally finished my homework and even then couldn't sleep, realizing there was one main command I would have to voice in every situation . . . and wondering if I had the courage to do it. Tomorrow knew the answer.

THE PAGES OF the ER logbook filled quickly as the desert sun rose; we were hit with patients early and often. The first few were like being home—dehydration, migraine headache, and a kidney stone, cases caused by the heat of the desert and that would become repetitive over the course of the summer. I was nervous, but hid it well. A few jokes here and there, busting Major Boutin over his choice of Cherry Walnut as the coffee of the day; even on the walk over to the hospital Rick said I still "looked like shit but at least had a dynamic stride." I didn't even know that he knew the word "dynamic." My thoughts of Rick's vocabulary were interrupted by a medic's tap on the shoulder.

"Word from Warhorse, sir. They're sending an overdose by chopper."

"What? Overdose?" I was trying to ready myself for gunshot wounds and blown-off limbs, but hardly expected I'd be treating a soldier who ODed.

"Forward base Warhorse, sir, about an hour up the road. I'll give Major Villines a heads-up."

Todd Villines was the only cardiologist in Iraq and was stationed at our CSH. Regular Army from Walter Reed, he didn't travel with our group of reservists. His expertise was caring for complex medical cases. But I wasn't thinking about him or Warhorse. I was wondering, *Overdose?*

When the chopper landed and the doors to the ER blew inward, the bluest human I had ever seen was having CPR done. *Jesus, whatever he took killed him.* I took a deep breath, fingered my cheat cards listing resuscitation protocols, and went to work. Shock to the chest, breathing tube inserted, heart drugs administered—I didn't need to look anything up, and best of all didn't act like a frozen statue.

After ten minutes of sweat, I finally had the time to take a big-picture view of the patient. Just a kid. His ID said twenty-one years old, and who knows what he put into his system and why.

"Man, he is one dark shade of blue."

I looked up, it was Dr. Villines.

"Know what he took?" he asked.

"No clue. I do know the tube is in the right place and pumping in lots of nice fresh O_2. Heart is now beating on its own with a stable rhythm but he's still blue as a berry."

"No kidding, he looks like a Smurf." Villines's eyes flickered from chart to patient to me. "Good job, Dave. Let's get him over to the ICU."

And with "good job" ringing in my ears, I walked back to my desk. Pulling a picture of my kids from my wallet, I thought about the Smurf. Does his mom or dad carry a snapshot of him in their wallet? Do they know what he just did and how close he came to needing a casket? And with that dark blue shade, he still wasn't out of the woods. Some scattered pieces of information from his unit suggested the overdose was intentional—the kid recently broke up with his girlfriend. Lab tests would later tell us what pills were sucked down to do the job.

I stood up to head outside for some fresh air and was nearly bowled over by a group of medics sprinting toward the landing pads. I never even heard the bird until it was seconds from landing. A pivot and slow trot brought me back to Alpha bay.

"Gunshot wound on the way, sir. One litter." The medics prepped the bay for the casualty as I grabbed gloves, clear protective goggles, and fingered my index cards like a rosary.

"Who's first call for surgery?" I asked.

"Colonel Reutlinger."

"Please page him and give Dr. Stanton a heads-up. Let's get ready for some business, ladies and gentlemen."

The words flowed with a confidence I didn't feel. As the stretcher rolled in, several staff members closely followed, gawking and craning for a look at the wounds. *Hurry up, Rick*, I mouthed silently. *This is a trauma-palooza and I could use a hand.*

The patient was an Iraqi soldier, blown up by an IED, and then shot as he got out of the vehicle. Medics kept pace with the stretcher at perfect speed, cutting off clothes and giving me a report as the wheels revolved through small pools of blood.

"Multiple shrapnel wounds. Gunshot to left chest. Partial amputation right leg. BP 90/50, pulse 150, respirations 30. Ten milligrams of morphine on board."

I gave a quiet nod at Twomey as the stretcher came into the bay headfirst and my eyes went to the body writhing before me. There was blood everywhere and crooked splinters of bone where a leg used to be. *Easy as A-B-C, Dave.* I quickly scanned the patient and forced myself to ignore the missing leg. A snug tourniquet had that problem under temporary control, but the bone splinters lying upon a blood-saturated sheet were a magnet to the eyes.

Reciting my lessons aloud to Major Twomey, I followed the trauma protocol to the letter.

A. Airway intact and open. No obstruction.

B. Breathing—good breath sounds bilaterally. Trachea midline.

C. Circulation—skin warm. Heart sounds are clear. Capillary filling less than two seconds.

D. Deficits to neuro are none. Patient alert. Glasgow Coma Scale 15 of 15.

The voice coming from my mouth wasn't my own but Twomey scribbled the words onto the trauma log. I methodically moved around the stretcher. "How are our lines? Good ones? You guys are great. Check that tourniquet, please." *Keep it calm. Take your time.*

Next came a check of pulses, abdomen, and pelvic bones. My hands slid up and down every inch of what was left of the Iraqi's limbs. My fingers rose and fell over rough skin peppered with shrapnel, and the small bumps where the tiny pieces of metal hid just under the surface.

As I recited my findings, the noise level in the room seemed to rise to a dull incomprehensible rumble, just enough to keep us from hearing each other around the stretcher, and me from hearing myself think. I then felt the jostle of extra bodies coming to the stretcher to take a peek and a poke at the patient. I was now being pushed to the edge of the cliff and the ground below me was starting to crumble. I was going to lose control.

Looking up, I said, "I need everyone who isn't in this bay to button it up, and if I didn't ask you into the bay, please get out and get behind that red line." It was the order I had worried about, the new guy telling people to get out of his way. But it was an order of necessity; the only cure for chaos was calm, even a false calm. And I worried how it would be received coming from me. Today, the response from the uninvited was a wilted bouquet of looks—dirty, confused, and sour. But when I looked across the room at Rick and Bernard, both of whom were still waiting quietly on the spectator side of the red line, I got a pair of welcomed winks. I finished up my exam, gave a few medication orders, and stepped across the room as I snapped off my bloody gloves.

"Rick, I think this guy needs a look-see of the belly. Feels like some of that metal is deeper than it looks, he's a little on the rigid side. Hey, Bernard, waiting for the bus?"

"I just was wandering by when this helicopter tried to give me a haircut. Sweet Jesus. Nice job in there, man. Say, did you eat this morning?"

"Yes, Mom."

"And how much did we eat?"

"Enough, Mom." *God, the thought of food makes me want to retch.*

Next, I walked over to Bill Stanton, who also was patiently waiting his turn.

"Hey, Billy, I'm getting films of both femurs, maybe the left hand and wrist. Anything else right off the bat?"

"Dude, not from a distance. Finish up the real-doctor stuff, then I'll step in. I'm cool."

As the patient went off for a CAT scan and X-rays, I crawled to my desk, imitating a man who has just finished a marathon through the steaming jungles of the Amazon. I was spent and, I now noticed, sweat-soaked. *But the patient had survived, I had survived, and like an animal had staked out my turf.* I prayed it would be enough to get me through the bad days ahead.

End of shift came quickly. The only patients who came through were minor—at least for me. A shrapnel wound to the hand of an American who was able to walk in on his own after a helicopter ride, a guy who got his bell rung by an IED, as well as a potpourri of cuts, scrapes, and bellyaches. Rick came by to pick me up for dinner and we decided to stop by the ICU before chow to check on the Smurf. Todd had the ventilator settings pushed to the max, yet the kid was still a dark blue. *Not going to make it. Shit.* As we pushed open the doors to leave, the words came out of our mouths simultaneously: Let's stop and call home before we eat. Just a quick reassurance that our own kids are okay. The lines were short, the calls went quickly, and we left the phone tent with the temporary solace that our kids weren't fighting the battle to stay alive in a war zone.

Halfway through our $32 gourmet meal of dead pork chop in congealed gravy, Rick's beeper chirped.

"Looks like we've got a kid with a hot appendix. Want to help?"

It was a no-brainer. "You bet I do."

I looked forward to working a scalpel; more importantly, I was eager to see just what the OR was really like behind its mysterious blanketed entry. So far, my duties had been taking place in an ER that really wasn't too ugly or dirty, just red with blood and overflowing with tension.

The OR, on the other hand, was the great unknown of the hospital complex. The tents and containers that made up the operating rooms had literally been shipped by boat and constructed after we captured the base in the early months of the war. For me, the fifteen steps from the ER to the OR was the medical equivalent of a leap across the Grand Canyon.

We pushed through the dusty blanket and walked to the cheap plastic scrub sinks. A small push-pedal on the floor forced a miserly flow of water through the faucet. I mirrored Rick's every move, and tried to work my hands into a lather with the flimsy scrub brushes.

"Where are the scrubs?"

"Aren't any."

"Booties?"

"Aren't any."

"Lockbox for my pistol?"

"You're wearing it. C'mon, let's pop the hot tamale out of this kid's belly and go home. I bet we can do this in three minutes and thirty seconds. That's my record."

A thin set of doors with small plastic windows provided the last barrier between what was supposed to be a sterile operating room and the swirling dirt of the outside world. We swung them open with our elbows and hips, keeping our hands up and away in the classic surgical pose. Gown pulled on, gloves tugged over semiclean hands, and we were ready to cut. Almost.

"Hey, how about some music in here?"

The surgical tech replied, "What would you like to hear, Dr. Reutlinger?"

"How about some Billy Joe while we're working."

My eyes peered over my masked mouth and nose.

"Billy who?"

"Billy Joe. I got him on my iPod. Love him."

"You mean Billy Joe Bob Willie or some other hick?"

"No—B-i-l-l-y J-o-e! You know, like 'Piano Man' or something."

"You mean Billy JOEL, Rick?"

"That's what I said the first time. You deaf?"

By the time I rolled my eyes from the back of my head to the patient, Rick had already made the first incision and more. I'd never seen anyone surgerize so quickly, and so well. Skin, muscle, fascia, and peritoneum expertly sliced and separated.

"Now where is that little—?"

The sentence was interrupted by the sudden bang and rumbling boom of a nearby shell. The scalpel in Rick's hand swung up and cut through air, missing my biceps by an inch as the tiny OR shook and our legs staggered.

"What in hell's bells?"

"Rocket or maybe an IED just outside the gate, Colonel. Had to be close." It was the surgical tech, who'd been jostled by scores of similar blasts during his year-long deployment. He never flinched.

"Jeez, that'll wake the neighbors," Rick said.

The tech responded, "Want more anesthesia, Colonel?"

"No, thanks, I think I'd better stay awake for this one," came the nervous quip.

We were only a few hundred yards from the gate, far enough to be safe, close enough to be introduced to the limb-tearing blasts our troops challenged every day. A big breath later, we were back at work, faster than ever. I had a hard time keeping up, especially cutting the knots Rick speed-tied as the appendix was snipped out and the abdomen closed.

As I watched the express train of a surgeon zoom along, I realized, with the exception of the rattling blast, this operation was no different from any other. Tight quarters in a container, cheap plastic scrub sinks, packing a pistol—none of it mattered, or for that matter, was even noticed. My focus zeroed to a patient, a scalpel, and an abdomen. Once gloved and gowned, you were automatically transported into the mystical world known as surgery.

We left the OR a little wilted, and very tired as the twenty-hour

marathon of a day groaned to an end. We walked through the ICU
on our way out, silently staring at the still blue body of the Smurf,
chest heaving up and down as the respirator forced oxygen into his
unconscious lungs. *Damn.*

I don't know if we beat the record for the removal of an appendix
that evening, but I do remember the song that was blasting through
the room as we finished: "Only the Good Die Young."

7

THE TUG-OF-WAR

IT WAS YET another "first day," although this one would take place in darkness. I was finally scheduled for the night shift, which meant I had the whole day to kill before showing up for work at 7 P.M., or as my Army watch would say: 1900 hours. After more than a week of going to work in the light of day, this would be my first time working alone in the dark and loneliness of night, and I had to admit, I was more than a little skittish.

I was gradually getting used to the blood and gore of the ER and my confidence was rising steadily with each case that rolled through our doors. But when I worked the day shift, help was only footsteps away. At night, I would be the only doctor in the hospital, and without phones, my sole tether to help was the pagers my fellow doctors kept next to their pillows.

Although my buddies would be less than half a mile away snoring in their bunks, that half a mile would seem like a continent especially if a bird made a surprise landing or I had someone tank out in the ICU. The only three doctors with instant availability would be me, myself, and I, and the way I was feeling, that trio reminded me of the

Three Stooges. As I lay in bed waiting for my watch alarm to beep, all I heard was *Dr. Howard, Dr. Fine, Dr. Howard,* quickly followed by a cadence of *Dr. Hnida, Dr. Hnida, Dr. Hnida.*

I shook the chant out of my head and skipped down the stairs to pick up Rick. Like me, he had been wide awake for hours, reading, killing time, and watching mental reruns of the experiences of the last few days. I envied his ability to read. At home, I normally knocked off about two books a week—usually spy or adventure novels—but here I found I couldn't read more than a sentence or two before I had to put the book down. It was a loss I would carry the entire rotation, and I mourned not being able to mentally escape each night, even for a few minutes. Rick, on the other hand, was now reading some book that claimed God was dead, or maybe never existed in the first place. The thought creeped me out and our morning together started off with me calling him a perverse shithead.

By the time we made it to breakfast, most of the doctors and staff were already there, having a heated discussion over some obscure worthless piece of trivia. The game took place on a regular basis no prizes or reward, just the satisfaction that you knew something of no practical value. The morning's stumper was "What is Barbie's real name?" courtesy of Bill Stanton.

Answers and comments flew up and down the table as we raced against an imaginary clock.

"She's a fucking doll. How can she have a real name?"

"This is a bullshit question."

"I know this one, it's Barbie Mattel."

"Who cares? She's a little plastic doll with little plastic boobs."

Bill looked smugly at the group. "Barbara Millicent Roberts."

"You're on drugs, man."

"No way."

"Yes, gentlemen, Barbara Millicent Roberts. And she was born in 1959, which means Reutlinger might like to date her."

Rick shot back, "Yeah, well, what about Ken?"

From down the table: "Rick, she's make-believe, for Christ's sake."

With that, we carried our trays away and took off for the hospital.

Medical rounds were held every morning at 0730 in the Ortho offices just around the corner from the OR, and even though I wasn't formally scheduled to work until night, I still had to show up for morning rounds.

The exercise basically consisted of all the docs, head nurses, therapists, and psych people getting together to review the progress of the patients in the hospital, look at any interesting X-rays or CAT scans, and make sure no one had screwed up in the previous twenty-four hours. Most days things were fairly painless—the main pressure was making sure we got the wounded evacuated as quickly as possible, and getting the injured Iraqis out of the gate to the local hospitals. The latter was the pressure-filled job of Arabic-fluent liaisons who worked their buddy lists to try to find a family member or a friend who would assume the care of an Iraqi we wanted out the door. As far as the U.S. Medical Command in Baghdad was concerned, an empty hospital was a good hospital.

The numbers that day weren't bad, only seven patients. With a capacity of eight beds in the ICU, and twenty in what was called the intermediate care ward, we could hold twenty-eight, with a special lying-room-only section for overflow crowds if necessary. We didn't know it, but there would be days ahead when the "No Vacancy" sign lit up at the door to our CSH.

The first order of business was to review X-rays and scans. As we crowded around a small computer, images of splintered bones underlying mangled arms, legs, and hands lit up the screen—the kind of injuries none of us ever really saw back in the States. A few murmurs and holy shits cycled through the group. We then moved on to some CAT scan images, which still looked like Rorschach tests and mud puddles to me. The realization was a slap in the face; I was still a lost soul wandering aimlessly in CAT scan land and needed to hit the *CAT Scans for Dummies* book harder.

Rick's appendix kid was doing great, and would be out of the ward in another day. And stunningly, the Smurf turned pink in the predawn hours and would be weaned off the ventilator over the course of the day. First glances didn't show signs of brain damage; maybe the kid would luck out. In any case, his next stop would be the States and then legal charges and court-martial. As would be the case with most of our patients that summer, the former Smurf would soon be out of sight, out of mind; there simply wasn't time to dwell on former patients, at least not while we were constantly replenished with new.

The last American soldier on the agenda was one I hadn't seen or heard about, a young soldier with hysterical blindness. After one too many missions swerving IEDs, this guy lost his vision. It happened a few days before and the patient was flown in from an outlying post during the night. He claimed he couldn't see the hand in front of his face, and a bright light was only a shadow. That meant he had to be led by hand from the ICW to the latrine or to the sidewalk for a smoke. Last night, he said he wanted to be left alone while having a cigarette, and when his nurse walked away she peeked back as she rounded a corner and saw him bend over, pick up a stone, and toss it at a sign. He then flicked his butt on the ground, walked over, and ground the embers out with his heel. This twenty-four-year-old wasn't blind but was an everyday young man who had cracked under the stresses of war.

Now our eyes were blank and peering at the floor, confused, yet a little frustrated at the young soldier for taking up valuable resources and time, then, just as quickly, disappointed at ourselves for feeling anything but pity. He'd be shipped to Germany, and we'd never learn if therapy would fix him or if he'd be dodging mental bullets and bombs to the day he died.

We had a few "housekeeping" items to discuss before being dismissed, the most important of which was the rumor of a big offensive slated to start within days, or weeks, depending on the setting of the bullshit-o-meter. The Surge was beginning, and its opening act

would start with a bang. Although we minions weren't supposed to
know details, for fear we would leak the info by e-mail or phone, it
was important for the hospital to ramp up and be ready from a staffing and supply standpoint. But as far as we were concerned, it didn't
matter. There would be no extra doctors sent to help us—busy or slow
we would trudge to work and do our jobs each day.

After rounds, we ambled over to the ER for coffee, and were told
flight conditions were "red"—meaning there were swirling sandstorms
in the area and no copters would be flying. No business expected at
least for a few hours. Which meant it was time for the morning mati-
nee. The morning's feature film on someone's laptop was the medics'
favorite: *Kill Bill*. Male and female, the medics watched, and then
rewatched, testosterone-laden DVDs with the highest violence and
gore ratings.

I knew I couldn't go back and nap; Rick had little going on at
the moment, so we decided to hike down the road and check out
the PX, a small building that served basically as our little corner gro-
cery. We didn't need anything, but thought some window-shopping
might break up the day. The store seemed well stocked, especially
with essentials like toothpaste and deodorant—there was even hair
dye for the female soldiers on the base, as well as, I suppose, the vain
males who were showing a few gray strands. One aisle led to another,
and with each came an increasingly surprising item to be stocked in
a war zone. A great selection of CDs, DVDs, audio systems, video
games, and video game systems. For off-duty enjoyment on a not-
so-cool summer evening were barbecue grills and a variety of patio
furniture, even some with umbrellas. And to help you speed off into
the sunset, a separate trailer next to the PX, which housed an actual
All-American auto dealership. Not that there were any cars on the
lot, but you could sit and pick a sleek beauty out of a catalogue, get
financing on the spot, and have that baby waiting for you when you
hit the States at the end of your deployment. Just one more thing to
widen the chasm separating my war and that of my father's.

"What in the name of shit's sake is all of this stuff? Cars? Trucks?" I said to Rick.

"I guess it's to keep morale up."

"Hell, I've got a truck back home—I need one here. This gravel is kicking the shit out of my feet. My feet need morale, not me."

Which was true—the combination of heat, sweat, and suffocating boots worn twenty hours a day had caused an entire layer of skin to peel off my feet and every step on raw skinless soles felt like a walk across hot coals.

Hands on hips, Rick stared at the trailer. "Let's see if they've got any Harleys in there."

"No, thanks, I've satisfied my midlife crisis by joining the Army and coming here."

Curious, we went in to browse and kick some imaginary tires. The small office was staffed by a contractor with a clipped accent we couldn't quite pin to a location.

"May I help you gentlemen?" asked the contractor-salesman.

"I'd like to buy a car," I said.

"Excellent. And what precisely are you interested in?"

"Anything but brown. I'd lose it in this country. Good air-conditioning. And something fast—we've got places to go, people to see, soldiers to operate on."

Eyebrows raised, the salesman stared at us with the early symptoms of confusion. And I was just getting revved up.

"Plus these are new cars, right? You're not a used car salesman? You know what they say about them."

Turning, I looked at Rick.

"Can we trust this guy? I mean, he's got a good face."

Rick nodded thoughtfully and said, "I think so. He's so trustable, I'd even let him pick one for you. One other thing, though, a siren would be good."

"Excellent idea, Dr. Jekyll."

Turning back, I said, "Okay, so why don't you pick a winner for me and we'll come by, say a week from Tuesday, and pick her up."

The answer was a series of hems and haws.

"Uh, I don't think you understand, sir, the cars, uh, they are not here. You buy them today at a discount and then get the vehicle when you return home."

"But that really doesn't help me a bit," I said. "I don't have wheels here. And me and my friend here are old guys who need transportation."

"Dave, I think that's why the lot looked empty. I think the Army has let us down for the first time ever. Let's hit the road."

The bell above the door gave a small ring as we left.

I turned to Rick as we began our trek back to the hospital. "So tell me, man, is this why we're in this country? I never knew one of the perks of war was a new car."

"Who the hell knows? I could use a new pickup, though. Mine's got two hundred thousand miles on it."

As we walked, the ground began to shake with the vibrations of incoming medevacs. So much for condition red—the starter's pistol had been fired into the dissolving haze. The ER was abuzz with activity; Gerry Maloney was running today's show and had his hands full with IED-damaged limbs.

Rick and I both stepped in and eyeballed the less severely wounded men, but the bigger view showed three bays filled with ortho cases. Bill Stanton went from stretcher to stretcher, prioritizing the injuries and deciding who would need the knife or, today, the saw first.

A sandy-haired kid in his midtwenties quietly wept on his stretcher, knowing his mangled leg was hanging by a thin sinew of flesh at the knee.

"Please don't take my leg. God, please don't take my leg," he murmured.

In the chaos of a noisy room, Bill picked up the soldier's plea amidst the chatter, came to an abrupt stop, and walked straight to the crying soldier.

He knelt down to eye level and placed his hand on a soot-smeared forehead. In a soft voice whose words flowed with a gentleness that seemed foreign in a war zone, Bill comforted his new patient, lying helpless on a stretcher, forced to trust a man he'd hoped he would never meet.

"I'm Dr. Stanton, the orthopedic surgeon. I'm going to level with you and tell you your leg is in bad shape. But I promise you, I will do everything, *everything*, I can do to make it better. Dude, if there's any way I can fix it, I will do that."

His hand gently stroked the frightened soldier's head as tears leaked a path down the soot-covered cheeks.

"But you have to trust me, if it's better that your leg comes off to save your life, I'm going to do that. For you and for your family. I'm going to take really good care of you. I promise. So let's give you some medicine to take the pain away and help you relax."

The fear slowly melted off the soldier's face, but as Bill turned, it was devastating to see the price he had paid for speaking the words. Bill knew the leg was finished, and could probably remove what was left with a simple pair of scissors. He was being held prisoner by one of the new medical axioms of this war: lose the limb, save the life. As would be the case with stretchers filled with assaulted extremities this summer, Bill would decide that a young soldier alive with a good prosthetic was better than a young soldier sent home in a coffin. Bill looked like he had aged thirty years in the course of this one conversation, his face a foreshadowing of the horrible decisions we all would be forced to make this summer without time for deep contemplation or thought.

Wiped out from just surveying the carnage, I pitched in and helped out a scrambling Gerry, then walked back to my quarters for a quick nap before my evening shift. As I started to doze, my pager went off. *Shit. What do they need?* The pager simply read: "A controlled detonation will take place in fifteen minutes." Someone must have found an unexploded shell on the base, or an IED just outside the wire. The standard procedure for a "controlled det" was to blow it up before it could hurt someone, and it seemed like a good idea to give us all a warning so we wouldn't shit our pants when the base rumbled from the big bang. Now unable to doze, I sat on the edge of my bunk like it was New Year's Eve, watching the countdown tick away the fifteen minutes. Then when the moment came for the climax, there weren't any noisemakers besides the ever-present rumble of the generators and occasional helicopter buzzing the camp. Twenty minutes, thirty minutes, forty minutes—zip zilch nada. Thanks for the warning but how about delivering on the promise? Sleep was now out of the question. I headed over to the DFAC, grabbing a paper plate of dried-out ham-and-cheese sandwiches to provide some energy for the night ahead.

Gerry had done a nice job of clearing the place out, and as I locked away my pistol, he gave me the change-of-shift report.

"We've got an urgent litter with an ETA of twenty mikes. Sounds like an EPW with a GSW to the pelvis."

"So in English, we've got a bad guy shot in the gut coming in by chopper in about twenty minutes and he ain't walking in on his own two feet. Gerry, why do you insist on trying to fuck with my head?"

"Pure love and affection for a colleague as well as understanding the unique machinations of the military."

"Shit, Gerry, you love the Army so much, you probably carry pictures of it in your wallet."

Almost twenty minutes to the second, the doors crashed open with a hurrying bloodstained stretcher whose occupant had skin the color of wax paper. The rolling wheels left bloody tracks on the floor.

"Gunshot wound pelvis. BP 100/48. Pulse 140. Spontaneous respirations 36."

The flight medic's voice was rapid-fire and businesslike. As our staff went to work to secure IV lines and cut off clothing, he pulled me aside.

"This might be the asshole who planted the IEDs that got our folks this morning. They caught him digging some new holes in the same area and nailed him when he took off."

The rest of the story dissolved into a distant mishmash of words. The only thing I could hear was the voice from earlier in the day: "God, please don't take my leg." The echo of that voice mixed with the high-pitched moaning coming from our new patient. The bomber.

It was now our job to save the life of an insurgent who could have been the one who took out three of our GIs this morning, leaving them with mangled limbs and scarred faces. If they were lucky to survive our fast-food surgery, they faced a new life where every morning began with strapping on a fake leg and a look into a mirror that answered with a face that didn't look like the one they had left home with.

I turned and stared at my medics as they cut off clothing and hung IVs. Young kids. Should be home. Going to parties. Gorging on pizza. I tried to picture them in civilian clothes but all I could see was reality.

Sweat dripping into eyes. Nostrils flaring. Shallow panting breaths. They didn't look at who this guy really was—the enemy—they just knew he was a patient and did what they would do with any other patient.

My exam told me the insurgent was in bad shape and going down the tank rapidly; a couple of gunshot wounds to the pelvis and groin put him into the downward spiral of shock. We started pumping blood into him as fast as we could—American blood—then paged Rick and Bernard. They hustled over quickly from the barracks, took one look, and ordered the insurgent wheeled into surgery.

Their next looks were to me, an odd silent exchange. Here we were: American doctors dressed as American soldiers. We wear uniforms, carry weapons, and even salute when we have to. Now we faced the litmus test of our oaths: military versus Hippocrates. Tonight, as Rick and Bernard broke their gazes and strode toward the

OR, it was clear Hippocrates won, and though we didn't dwell on it at the time, so did American values. No flags waving, no rousing speeches, no Fourth of July fireworks—we just did what we had been trained to do.

I think we have an advantage as doctors. We go into auto mode, a skill we begin learning the first days of internship and residency. It's no longer a good guy/bad guy/I don't know what side he's on guy. We see bleeding—we see broken—we see things that need fixing.

That night, Rick and Bernard spent six hours trying to plug the leaks in an enemy pelvis made by American bullets. The X-rays on the OR viewbox didn't list nationality, the scalpel didn't cut differently into flesh that was hostile, and the blood pooling inside the pelvis was just as red as what flowed through our veins.

As Rick and Bernard tried to embroider together a torn-apart body, I worked away in the ER, caring for several guys whose truck had hit a roadside bomb. Their wounds weren't life-threatening, so when word filtered from the OR that my friends needed a quick extra set of hands, I left my American soldiers and scrubbed in for a short time. What kind of doctor walked away from his own GIs to try to save an enemy bomber?

As I pushed open the doors of the OR, I was greeted by the voice of Jimmy Ruffin softly playing in the background, asking what becomes of the brokenhearted?

The tune was accompanied by the steady beat of a heart monitor and the "whoosh-whoosh-whoosh" of the ventilator pushing a rhythmic flow of air into the insurgent's lungs. As I edged my way toward the table, I glanced at the bomber's pale and sickly face. On top of the pastiness sat the slightest wisp of a mustache.

"Where do you want me?" I asked.

Rick positioned me next to Bernard on the far side of the table, my main job being to suction pooled blood out of the depths of the abdomen. Besides the faint music in the background, there were few words heard. It was all business.

"Mayo retractor."

"Kelly clamp."

"Curved snips."

"Metzenbaum."

"Dave, shift to your left for a second, we got to get down in there. Can't see."

I pushed a step to the side and bumped into a body that wasn't supposed to be in my way. Before I could open my mouth, I realized it was our chaplain. She was bent over at the head of the OR table, her hand tightly grasping the limp hand of the insurgent. Through her mask, I could see the faint facial movements of her mouthing a prayer. I wondered who she was praying to. The God I believed in? Allah? Some generic Supreme Being? I guess it didn't matter. Our chaplain would come and hold the hand of any critical patient on the table; friend or foe, there was no distinction. She took the same approach as we physicians; it was a human being on the table, one that needed urgent medical or spiritual care. The right, wrong, or morality of it could be argued by others. Others that weren't in the room and standing in our bloody boots.

The case continued.

"Adson forceps."

"Sponge. No, give me two or three. Quick."

"More suction. C'mon, Dave, faster."

"Now tie that bleeder off. Atta boy."

As I watched Rick and Bernard move in concert, it seemed like they'd worked together for decades. They were maestros in the OR; I, on the other hand, was tone-deaf. But their patience with me was infinite.

After twenty units of American blood and buckets of American sweat, Rick and Bernard closed the abdomen and pelvis. It looked like the IED planter might make it.

As I walked through the blanketed door of the OR, I saw the first peek of dawn. Almost twenty-four hours had passed since I lay in my bunk dreading my first night shift, a shift that turned out much differently than I expected. Things moved so quickly that instead of fear, my biggest battle was one of ethics. I cleared the remaining soldiers out of the ER and met up with Rick and Bernard at the chow hall for a meal the clock said was breakfast.

They were silent except for occasional spurts of exhausted anxiety. We all hated the guy for what he had done to our soldiers, yet the conversation kept on drifting into a weird doctor-speak of "I hope that oozing stops" and "that left kidney did not look good" followed by "those retroperitoneal tears are a bitch" and "I'll go back and check on him, you go to bed." I know they replayed the surgery over and over in their heads, just like all good doctors do.

The insurgent survived the dawn—due in large part to our ICU nurses—but later that morning started to bleed again. No matter how many units of blood and blood products he got, his body was shutting down. He needed to go to surgery again.

This time I scrubbed in with Rick and Bernard from the start. They had done a helluva job putting together the jigsaw puzzle that was once a functioning abdomen. Yet no matter what, when a person's blood stops clotting, there is nothing more you can do. The insurgent went into cardiac arrest three times on the table, and three times we shocked him back to life. Yet it wasn't enough. There was nothing left to sew, because with every stick of the needled suture, a fresh flow of blood began.

We were witnessing the "rude unhinging of the machinery of life"—a phrase coined during the Civil War to describe the process of a body rapidly going into shock, a condition where blood ceases to clot, blood pressure plummets, and the heart exhausts itself to a standstill. Throughout the ages, countless physicians have stood by helplessly as their patients spiraled down the pathway to death; there was nothing they could do to halt the journey. We reluctantly joined that centuries-old fraternity.

It was time to close up the abdomen and come up with plan B.

But we knew plan B didn't exist for this insurgent. He died about thirty minutes later despite the best care we had to offer.

At the foot of his bed in the ICU, the three of us quietly stood pondering his limp body, shaking our heads slowly as we tried to figure out why he planted the IED in the first place. He probably needed a few bucks for his family—we heard the going rate for shoveling a hole was $20 a dig. I stared at the adolescent attempt at a grown-up mustache.

Our insurgent was just fifteen years old. I know my thoughts drifted toward home—and distant stares told me Rick and Bernard went to theirs, and to our own kids who were once fifteen years old. When the worst they did was get home a few minutes late on a Friday night. They didn't plant bombs. They weren't the enemy. This kid was.

We just walked away, not saying a word. Our steps out of the ICU mirrored those of old men.

I walked to the latrine to shave off a day's growth of stubble. I stared into the mirror, rubbing on a thick lather of Barbasol, not sure whether it was good that a bad person had died or sad that *this* bad person had died.

After what I had done, I wasn't sure I liked the face I saw in the mirror, then, too, neither did I hate it. At least I was able to look and face myself.

8

"A PICTURE IS
WORTH A THOUSAND TEARS"

IT WAS A bustling day in the ER when an unannounced chopper thundered in carrying a young soldier whose vehicle was blown ten feet into the air by a well-hidden IED. His condition was one step past critical by the time he got to me. I had to ignore the raw stumps that minutes before were a complete arm and leg; tourniquets were on snugly and the oozing could wait. There was no time to waste before fixing the more important blood pouring from his neck, as well as trying to figure out why his abdomen was rapidly swelling like a balloon.

To look at his face, though, you would have thought life was fine. There was no sign of damage, just little smudges of dirt on his cheeks and peacefully closed eyes. With short-cropped blond hair and a square jaw, he reminded me of a typical twentysomething I would see in my practice for a winter's sore throat or a sprained ankle from a summer evening softball game. But that's where the resemblance came to an end. From the neck down, this kid was in bad shape. The force of the blast had ruptured his liver and spleen and I was squirming as I gazed at the small holes burned into his neck by hot chunks of shrapnel. I had no clue where these holes led and what the hot shards of metal had hit as they ripped through the skin and deeper tissues. I shut out images of home and the faces I'd left behind. Forcing myself into medical autopilot, I went to work trying to keep the soldier alive.

It took twenty-eight minutes of medical improv to get him stable enough for surgery. We made up treatments as we went along; pumping in countless units of blood and vials of medications, cautiously peeking under, then changing saturated bandages, and adjusting tubes and dials to force oxygen into his reluctant lungs. I was soaked with his blood by the time we were done, but it would be hours until I could shower and change my uniform. The warm stickiness didn't bother me, though, and even served an important purpose: reminding me there was a young man who belonged to that blood, and now he belonged to me. I was so tired I was weaving on my feet, but there was no way I could abandon this soldier.

Rick was the surgeon on that day, and since I was finishing my ER shift, I scrubbed in to lend a hand. We spent six hours doing patchwork surgery to keep this kid alive, and by the time we tore off our gloves and gowns, he was barely hanging on by that dreaded medical term: a thread. The worst injury was a small, impossible-to-find blood vessel, leaking at the base of the skull. We just couldn't get to it; all we could do was hope the leak would just gradually clot over and stop bleeding. He was too unstable to put on a plane to Germany or the States for more extensive repairs, so the battle shifted to a hand-wringing waiting game. Rick and I trudged out of the OR, leaving the young soldier in the ICU nurses' able hands, too bummed out to say a word, with nothing left to do but hope he took a turn for the better and made it onto one of the nightly flights to Landstuhl or Walter Reed.

The surgery was tough, but the next task was even tougher; Rick volunteered to go outside into the dark heat and talk to the soldiers in the kid's unit. Bearing the bad news is the most painful job a doctor has, and this task seemed to carry extra hurt. There would be tears, slumped shoulders, walls punched in anger. I just sank my head in depressed exhaustion and shuffled down the walkway, as Rick trudged in the opposite direction toward an anxious group of battle-dirtied warriors. He was hurting and so was I, but we couldn't show that hurt to anyone besides each other. Often here, a projected "never say die" attitude really meant "we're futilely trying to cheat death." We needed to hold each other up as we staggered down the thin line separating life and death.

Sad and lonely, I thought of my family. This was one of those times all I wanted to do was hold my children tight and never let go. All four of mine were right around the ages of most of the soldiers I cared for, and every time a chopper dropped from the sky, I whispered two prayers: *God, thank you it's not one of my kids coming on that bird*; then quickly, *Please help me save the kid who's coming in, the one who belongs to some other parent.* It was true, every turn of the blades of a medevac caused my heart to ache for someone . . . including myself.

The bright lights of the ER snapped on as I walked through the doors, interrupting the small crowd of medics watching a DVD. For the first time in days, the place was quiet. Eerily so. The medics flipped off the movie and scurried toward me.

"What's the word, sir? Is he gonna to make it? You guys were in there for a long fucking time."

All that came out was a soft mumble, "Man, I don't know. He's oozing and bleeding from everywhere. His neck is Swiss-cheesed. But he's hanging tough."

Our chief nurse took a tentative step toward me.

"Uh . . . well, sir, when we cut his pants off his wallet fell on the floor. You ought to take a look."

I shouldn't have taken a look.

Right inside the fold of the sweat-stained wallet was a photo of the soldier and his family. He had a bright, bubbly wife with arms around two kids dressed up in their Easter best, the boy about three years old and the little girl about a year and a half. All smiling. All happy. All together.

Now things were too personal. The picture looked exactly like the ones my family took every Easter. I couldn't stop picturing my kids on respirators with missing limbs and holes in their necks. Then came snapshot images of teenagers lying on a sidewalk after being shot while fleeing a school. I shook my head back and forth, violently trying to get the images the hell out of my brain. What was going on here? I usually did a good job blocking out personal details when a life was on the line, it was the only way to ensure the psych bell didn't toll for me. That's why I made it a rule *not* to look at the names of those soldiers teetering on the line between life and death. They were "the leg," "the pelvis," or in this case, "the neck." As I sank down at my homemade plywood desk to do the paperwork on the case, I avoided looking at this soldier's name. I DID NOT want to know it. But unfortunately, I did. He was "Honey" and "Daddy." And I was one step from losing my sanity. The photo had blown a giant hole in my protective armor.

Each day, we got up, shook out our boots and uniforms to dislodge any nighttime visitors from the neighborhood scorpion or spider families, strapped on our pistols . . . and our most important piece of a combat doctor's protective gear: mental armor. Only then could we head off and face whatever the medevacs were going to deliver to our front door. That morning had been no different, but I hadn't seen one of the worst days of my deployment coming. I never had the chance to add that extra layer of armor.

From the ER, I walked the quarter mile of sand back to my room in total darkness; my only companion the ever-present hot desert wind, whistling at me, mocking me for my weakness. The wind was right; I sucked as a doctor and was going to lose a young soldier because I wasn't good enough.

Back at my barracks, I showered for ten minutes longer than the mandated two, watching blood swirl down the drain until the water flowed clear. I felt I'd never truly wash his blood off my skin, just like I could never get the pungent odor of charred flesh to leave my nostrils; they were my scars of his battle. I finally tumbled into bed, stuck my iPod earbuds in, and turned on my nightly sleep aid, the sound of ocean waves. Tonight, though, even the rhythm of gentle surf couldn't keep me from reliving every slice of the scalpel and the tying of every stitch. What could we have done better? Though part of me knew that the honest answer was nothing, when it's your husband or dad on the table, that's just not good enough. After three nightmarish hours of trying to rest, I lurched my sleep-hungry body down the stairs and rapped on Rick's door.

"How'd you sleep, Ricky?"

With red-rimmed slits for eyes, he wearily answered, "Like crap. Harry was up all night. Billy went out at three for something. Heard a bunch of choppers. I think I had to piss six times. But no pages on the kid. That's good, but I couldn't stop thinking about the damn oozing from that neck. Let's go eat, then check him. I don't think I had any dinner last night."

He paused as he laced his boots.

"So who's the DS of the day?"

DS. Designated Saluter. Most of the doctors outranked everyone on the base, so a half-mile walk could easily have us returning three dozen salutes. To ease the strain on our arms and foreheads, we took turns walking one half step ahead of each other so at least one of us could make it to the DFAC, the chow hall, in peace.

With the best smirk I could muster, I replied, "You are, o great son of Oklahoma. And the salute of the day is the . . . Boy Scout."

Five minutes and twenty three-fingered Boy Scout salutes later, we made it to the DFAC for our typical breakfast of champions: powdered eggs, rock-hard bagels, and in Rick's case, four odd-looking, soggy excuses for grapefruits. He had restarted the infamous "Mayo

Clinic Grapefruit Diet," which Rick claimed could peel off twenty pounds in two weeks or less. You eat a ton of grapefruit for breakfast and lunch, then have an all-you-can-eat, anything-you-want dinner, and voilà, off comes the fat! The only problem is, the Mayo Clinic says the diet is bullshit, which explained why Rick hadn't lost an ounce in the month he'd been following it.

I told him, "You're a moron. The 'MD' behind your name stands for Moron Doctor. Does your wife know you're doing this?"

My tirade against Rick stalled as the rest of our crew staggered in and sat down at our table. It turns out we had gotten more business, in the form of a couple of guys who ran into an IED during the night. Bernard had to play bobbing for shrapnel in some guy's arm and leg for a couple of hours, after which Wild Bill pinned together a couple of fractures. Nothing too serious.

These wounded Americans would be fine and on a plane out of here that night, but would our guy be on it, too? Did his wife get the news yet? What was the family doing now as they waited for more information? The questions ate a hole in my brain.

A quick and fortunate shift in conversation led to current events and the topics of the day, as well as the ritual passing of the bottle. Tabasco. Down the line it went, splashing its way onto eggs, sausage, toast, biscuits, even Captain Walters's cornflakes. The banter was like a rapid-fire game show as we moved from one end of the table to the other.

First up was Sergeant Everson. "Best way to win the war is send Cheney on a hunting trip with the insurgents. That is fact, gentlemen."

Staring at the news on the closed circuit TV, Walters was next: "Scooter Libby gets pardoned. How come no one pardons me for my gas?"

My turn. "I've got some great ideas on how we can wrap this whole thing up and go home. So how come Petraeus won't return any of my calls?"

Rick sliced back, "You shouldn't have sneezed when you were doing his vasectomy."

Even with a mouthful of cereal, Bernard had something to say. "Did Bush do any LSD at Yale? Maybe we're here because he's having some weird flashbacks or something. I mean, this whole place is like a bad acid trip."

Bill Stanton decided it was his turn for a morning ballbust: "Rick, do you shit whole grapefruits or just wedges?"

The jokes were as lousy as the food, but we needed the laughs to help us cope with what we'd seen the night before and recharge our emotional batteries for what we'd face in the day ahead. We finished up and took off into a world filled with swirling sand particles so dense they threatened to block out the sun. Mouths shut tight and scarves wrapped around our noses, we snapped on goggles to keep our corneas from being sand-blasted and scarred.

The trek from the DFAC took more than its usual three minutes, delayed by saluting and dodging smoke-belching Humvees and gun trucks headed out on the day's missions. No one said it, but we were all hoping the same thing: that the number that went out would be the same that came back, and that no one would be making the return trip via medevac.

We cleared our weapons of ammo, double-checked the safety levers, and entered the hospital "complex" through a small break in the massive concrete blast walls. Rick and I headed straight to the ICU, closely followed by the rest of the doctors. We were thankful for any brilliant thoughts they might have, but more importantly for the support we felt from them just tagging along. We were a tight group: when anyone had a bad case, we all had a bad case. It was shared suffering.

Our kid was still alive, barely, but alive nonetheless. The ICU nurses, whom we called the "Angels of Mercy," had spent the night keeping him comfortable: cleaning him up, combing his hair, and talking to him. I always wondered if the near dead could hear; it was clear that the Angels didn't even consider it a question. They just whispered and spoke to the patient as if nothing was wrong, while the rest of us hid our fears and helplessness by playing the role of tough, unflappable doctors. We made busy looking at vital signs, respirator settings, and medication dosages. Then my eyes met the small table next to the bed. There sat the family snapshot, placed right in the direct line of sight of the soldier on life support. I bit my lip so hard it bled, but was saved when someone said we needed to get moving to make it to rounds on time.

The numbers this particular day weren't too bad. Besides a few Iraqis, we had the two soldiers in from the IED blast during the night, two Americans in the noncritical ward because of constipation-induced abdominal pain, another American with pneumonia, then our kid in the ICU. We crowded into a tight circle, which grew even tighter when it was time for Rick to explain our case, what we had done, and the prognosis: bad. The only thing we could do was watch, wait, and bite our nails.

"This GI is in bad shape. We can't fly him. He's still oozing and leaking from somewhere deep in the neck. It's coming from the base, in the back, right at the spinal cord. I can't see where. Dr. Stanton cleaned up the blown-off arm and leg. Dave and I did the best we could with the abdominal wounds. That part's stable. We'll watch him for a few more hours, then see if we need to go back in for that leak."

You could see a lot of eyes peering at the floor before we quickly moved on to three Iraqi patients who had decided to take full advantage of our hospitality.

By then, most of us had blocked out the chatter about the Iraqis and were mentally back in the ICU, standing over the bed of our most critical patient. The pressure drove us toward a rapidly approaching breaking point; we needed a laugh or else we'd cry. Our deliverance came in the unexpected form of a wounded Iraqi policeman with the name of Mohammed Focker. Which meant the next words out of Quick's mouth were, "So how is Mr. Focker this morning? When is he out of here?"

Since "Mo Focker" was an ortho case, a straight-faced Bill Stanton formally answered, "Sir, Mr. Focker is doing well. His fractured humerus is healing and Dr. Reutlinger has signed off the case since the gunshot wound is now closed over. We are simply waiting for disposition to his family or an outside facility."

That statement was met with a spontaneous chorus of "Focker! Come on, get that Focker out of here, we need the bed!"

Dr. Quick: "What about Focker's family?"

A quick refrain from the medical choir: "Yeah, what about Dom Focker or Woody Focker!"

Poor Mo. He was actually a very pleasant man and cooperative patient who had absolutely no idea his name was oh-so-close to an American profanity that got wheels of its own from a popular Hollywood movie. Little did he know his name brought our dark day a few minutes of light.

As rounds drew to a close, I snuck out to check the action in the ER. My shift actually started at seven, but I usually let the nurses and medics run the show for the first hour of my shift and only page me if there was a big problem. This day, the page came early. At 7:50, we got a static-filled radio call from "Badblood," the medevac unit that flew in the wounded. The wording was terse: two urgent litters/ multiple GSW/head, which, translated, meant two soldiers in critical condition coming in on stretchers with gunshots to the head. The medics went to work setting up the trauma bays with IVs and other equipment. The lab was called and told to warm up some blood. The OR was put on alert. And pages were sent out to the day's surgeons, Rick and Bernard.

We weren't given an estimated arrival time so I just told the crew to take off in shifts to the latrines, empty their bladders, and run back if they heard the choppers coming in. Since our whole hospital shook with a landing, an arrival was impossible to miss.

Ten minutes passed, then twenty. When the clock on the wall hit thirty, we started wondering what might be up, hoping the birds weren't involved in any firefights. Finally, at a nerve-stretched fifty minutes, we heard the whomp-whomp of the blades. Our medics sprinted out with their stretchers to the landing pad . . . then calmly walked back in, accompanied by two *walking* soldiers with *hand* injuries. I let my intestines return to the inside of my body and got out of the medics' way. It was always good news when the injuries were minor compared to what you dreaded they were going to be.

The two patients had been in a small firefight; though I'm not sure it's ever fair to call a firefight small, especially when the bullets are aimed at you. These two guys were scared and needed a little TLC and a joke. The joke was key, since it let a wounded guy know he was going to be okay. And a joke was my weapon of choice in defending myself from the horrors of the war, especially when I had a young one slowly bleeding to death in the ICU, but still needed to take care of other patients.

I typically took off my uniform top when I worked, simply wandering around in a T-shirt, with a nice little nametag made of surgical tape . . . by order of the hospital administrator.

"Major, I know it's hot and you can get bloody in that job of yours, but you need to wear a nametag so we know who you are and you look professional."

I thought the stethoscope was all I needed to make me authentic, but using a surgical tape nametag did allow me to change identities quicker than Superman. I could be anyone as long as the brass didn't catch me. Major Whiner. Major DeZaster, Major Jack Cass.

Today was a slam dunk.

"Good morning, gentlemen. I am Dr. Petraeus. I see you both have been given some lead injections by our friends, the enemy. Doesn't look too bad. We'll give you something for pain. Take some X-rays. You'll then get a visit from Iraq's favorite orthopedic surgeon if the bones are hit, otherwise we'll just clean you up and give you a nice comfortable bed to spend the night."

The nervous soldiers' eyes went even wider.

One blurted, "Did you say Dr. Petraeus? Like, are you related to the *General* Petraeus?"

"Yes, I am his father," I answered solemnly. "Say, have you ever seen *Star Wars*? You know Darth Vader and Luke Skywalker? Well, it's not like that for us. We get along great and never sword-fight. Now let's fix you guys up."

The soldiers were chuckling as the wheelchairs took them away for some X-rays in the nearby radiology tent. I sat down to drink, and then spit out, a cup of the morning's coffee: Pumpkin Spice. Who drinks this kind of stuff—especially in a war? And what idiot thought up Pumpkin Spice? Instead, I grabbed a Red Bull from the mini-fridge. A few minutes later, the two dinged soldiers returned from X-ray, feeling no pain from the morphine we had loaded them with before the trip. The films looked clean and the wounds superficial. Good news. All they needed was a "wash-out"—basically a power wash of the bullet holes—and a clean dressing.

As they were being wheeled away to the ward, one babbled in a drug-induced fog, "Doc, say hi to your son the general when you see him."

I laughed. "My pleasure. You can expect your medals within two weeks, sooner if they come UPS. May the Force be with you."

Okay, it was an insane asylum, but it was *our* insane asylum. Designed to make the soldiers feel at home while away from home and allowing us to act like nuts to keep from going nuts. And we needed that 24/7, because no sooner had the chuckles stopped than we heard a whomping sound and felt the ER start to vibrate. Another chopper. No warning, no heads-up.

This time when the medics sprinted out, they sprinted back in, pushing a stretcher occupied by an Iraqi policeman spurting blood in all directions. And the medics were doing CPR. Shit. My surgeons had left. The anesthesia people were busy and nowhere to be seen.

I went to Alpha bay and took my place at the head of the stretcher as the medics jostled into their assigned areas around the wounded soldier. It quickly became a contest to see who wouldn't puke first. He had no jaw. It was gone. Blown off. Yet he was still alive. There was a collective swallow of bile as we all kicked into our personal auto modes. I had seconds to get an airway in to help this poor guy breathe. Blindly probing with my finger, bubbles soon appeared from the middle of the bloody mass of unrecognizable flesh, and I found what used to be a mouth.

"Guys, I think we've got one good shot at this. Get me some suction. Hold him steady now." In went the airway tube—sliding smoothly along my finger, down the throat, and into the windpipe. Pure luck.

A medic grabbed my stethoscope and listened to the lungs.

"Good breath sounds both sides, sir. Very nice."

The medics got their IV lines in and poured in fluids and blood. X-ray came and shot a series of films. We watched as his blood pressure climbed and the patient began to stabilize. He might actually have a chance.

Now I asked for more details. "Who is this guy?"

The chief nurse answered, "Iraqi police."

"What's the story?"

"No clue."

I wanted to get him to a reconstructive specialist before something went wrong and he tanked on us, and told the chief nurse, "What do you say we get Balad on the line and spin up a bird to get this guy on the road? Time to say hi and goodbye."

Twenty minutes later the "Man Without a Face" was on his way. Odds were the docs at Balad would jigsaw-graft back together a human face. I'd seen their work and it was good. Our time with the patient was just twenty-eight minutes, and we'd never see him or his new face again.

As the medics swabbed the blood from the floor, I snuck out to sneak a peek at our kid in the ICU. Rick and Bernard were hovering like nervous parents.

Rick was somber. "Look at that blood. Still leaking. Pressure is dropping. We've gotta go back in, Bernard."

Bernard stood staring at the bandage that was soaking red. "You're right man. Need a hand?"

"Twenty, if you've got them."

Rick looked up, saw me at the foot of the bed, and said, "Dave, we could use you, too."

I answered quickly, "I'm in. Let me get someone to cover the ER."

I paged Mike to see if he could take over for a few hours. While I waited, it was back to work seeing patients. Fortunately, there weren't many waiting, which was unusual, and those who were waiting had problems just like the ones I typically saw back home. One guy who strained his back lifting a bag of something, another with a headache, then one other with chest pain. The one with chest pain was only twenty-two years old, so I wasn't too worried about heart problems. Nonetheless, I had the medics do the million-dollar workup: EKG, chest X-ray, lab work, the whole nine yards.

The headache guy was simple. A migraine, which was typical for guys working in 130-degree temperatures and not getting enough fluids. He needed a little pain medication to take the edge off and a lot of IV fluids to refill his tank.

As I worked my way to the next stretcher to see the patient with back pain, the train pulled in to the station, filled with a group of soldiers who had hit a small IED an hour before. Nothing too serious at first glance, but they all needed to be checked and cleared before being sent back to duty. There were five of them, so that was going to take some time.

I told one of the medics to tell the guy with back pain it might be a few minutes before I could see him.

The young specialist stammered, "But, sir, he's a sir."

Puzzled, I asked, "Meaning . . . ?"

He continued to stammer. "A colonel. And he says he's in a hurry. All he wants is some Vicodin."

With sprouting irritation, I quickly responded, "Tell the colonel to take a number. I don't give narcotics without an exam. And I need to see the IED guys before anybody else."

"He's really pissed, sir."

I could feel myself getting hot.

"Then give him a urinal."

We now had a full house and I was squirming for Mike to show up so I could hustle over to surgery in time. I made my way down the rows of stretchers once more.

The IED guys weren't in too bad shape; some ringing ears, a couple of headaches, and one bloodied eardrum whose owner couldn't hear very well. As I looked at the ruptured eardrum with my otoscope, I was blasted by a shouting voice less than an inch away from my face.

"I AM FINE, SIR. JUST A LITTLE HEADACHE. MY EAR HURTS BUT NOT TOO BAD."

Fighting the need to shout back, I evenly replied, "Okay, you don't have to yell. I can hear you just fine, even if you can't hear me very well."

"WHAT DID YOU SAY?"

"I said we captured Osama, the war is over, and we can all go home now."

"I'M FINE, SIR. JUST A LITTLE HEADACHE. MY EAR HURTS BUT NOT TOO BAD."

That clinched it. My young ruptured eardrum bought himself a night in our medical hotel.

Looking into his confused eyes I said, "Son, welcome to Paradise

General Hospital. You will be our guest for the night and you will not go back to duty until you can hear every single syllable I utter."

For good measure, I wrote it all down for him to read. He was going to be fine, but he wasn't going anywhere until we were sure he was fine. Too many concussions and head injuries had been missed or ignored, and none of us wanted a soldier to carry home the scourge of a hidden brain injury. When it came to IED blasts, we were cautious to the max, even if it pissed off commanders who were short-handed on troops to send out on missions.

My motherly ways were rudely interrupted by a whining screech from a couple of stretches down the line.

"I need someone here NOW!"

The asshole colonel.

I took my time strolling to his stretcher. As I pulled back the curtain, I told myself to be calm.

"Yes, Colonel, what can I do for you?"

"I need to get back to my office and get some work done. I don't need to be wasting my time sitting here waiting all day," he barked.

"Well, sir, maybe we can get the official war referees to call a time-out," I responded calmly, "you know, take a little break from the game so we can all catch up. Maybe we can make a phone call or something to the people in charge."

His face turned bright red and the veins on his forehead took on a dangerously explosive appearance.

"Wise guy, huh? MAJOR."

I now answered through gritted teeth, "No, doctor-guy, COLONEL. And I've got five guys who hit an IED in line ahead of you. And I know your back had a fight with your duffel bag, but they get to go first. Rule of the hospital. Rule of my ER."

He continued to push me to the edge with a sternly toned, "Well, hustle it up. I don't have all day."

Bowing at the waist, I quickly backed away from the stretcher.

"Yessir, yessir, yes—sir."

I would now go sweep the sidewalks and take out the trash before I'd examine him. Important rule: Never piss off the staff of an emergency room, or any medical office for that matter. It made me wonder what this self-important desk jockey would think about our young trooper who was slowly dying, one drop at a time. The one whose blood still stained my boots.

As I walked away cursing under my breath, Bernard came in.

"We're in a holding pattern. Bill is sticking a rod in some guy's tibia and then has to clean up a wound graft. Dude says he's hurrying."

I shook my head and pictured the steady drip from the unknown leak in the kid's neck.

"All right—just let me know. I'll be here. How's the kid doing?"

"Sinking. I think Rick is taking this one hard. Man, we're all taking this one hard. Even the Angels are hovering extra close. Shit, that leak is going to do the kid in. He's going to die no matter what, but we've got to try something."

Die no matter what. Damn, I didn't need Bernard to confirm what I already believed.

I looked over at the clock. Eleven A.M. here, which meant the middle of the night back home. Was his wife up? She had to have gotten word by now. I thought about what went through her mind as the pair of soldiers came to her front door to give her the news her husband was critically wounded. She probably didn't want to open the door because she knew why soldiers in dress uniforms travel in pairs to the homes of soldiers. The neighbors watch in sadness, yet are secretly relieved the soldiers passed by their houses.

She had no idea about us, a group of doctors—strangers thousands of miles away, feeling crushed by the pressure of fighting a battle destiny told us we would lose. We couldn't eat, couldn't sleep, and couldn't get our minds off her husband. I wonder if she knew how much we really cared? How the Angels hover around his bed, talking to him about his beautiful children, and making sure he is comfortable? And what about those kids? They'd never see their dad again, but they didn't know it yet. The waiting, that dreaded and powerless unknown, is one of the greatest tortures a soul can ever know.

Once again, I flashed back to Littleton. The night of the shootings, scores of parents were herded to a nearby elementary school, waiting as the authorities sorted through long lists of missing students. Who was found at a friend's or neighbor's house, who was wounded and in the hospital, and who wasn't on either list. Those not on a list were still lying in the school. Vibrant teens who left for school that morning, like any morning, now lifeless under desks and tables. The frightened look in the eyes of a parent waiting for news, but dreading it.

What did the eyes of our soldier's wife look like? Sleepless, red, and tear-stained, filled with dread and anxiety as she waited for word that lay in our helpless hands. Seven thousand miles away and we couldn't comfort her, couldn't reassure her, couldn't hold her hand and tell her we were going to try somehow to make everything right. The questions and images racing through my exhausted mind were making me nuts.

Just then, Mike came strolling in and saved me from myself.

"Sorry, Dave, I was out running when my pager went off. Where do you need me?"

I gave him the colonel. Begged him to take the colonel, just to get the guy out of the ER. He was a bad vibe for all of us. In the meantime, I took off to check out the rest of the IED guys, while the medics went to work on a couple of new arrivals: a bellyache from desert-induced constipation and a badly cut hand belonging to some guy from the motor pool. The cases were quickies the medics could handle, and I could just sign off after a swift double-check of their work.

I shot a quick glance at the clock once again—twenty more minutes had disappeared. I fast-walked to the ICU to check the kid. The Angels surrounded his bed, doing busywork as they waited for the

OR to open up, while I tried to look at the big picture so I wouldn't see the family picture. Things weren't pretty. Blood pressure continuing to drop, and blood coming out as fast as we could transfuse it in. Logic told us to call it quits, but we couldn't. If we didn't pull out every single stop, every sleeve-hidden trick, and then invent a few more, we'd never be able to look in a mirror again. It all boiled down to the simple matter of why we were here and why we practiced the way we did: if it were our son or daughter in that bed, we would want everything possible done. Everything. As I turned to leave, I saw a tear trickle down the cheek of the head nurse.

I walked back into the ER, knowing I had to pull myself together. There were other patients to be seen, and if any of them were my son or daughter, I would want the doctor caring for them without distraction.

The tests on the young chest pain patient were all normal. It was a minor-league pulled muscle, but he needed some major-league convincing. With shaking hands and darting eyes, he begged for reassurance. "Are you sure it ain't my heart? My dad had a heart attack last year. I'm afraid to go to sleep."

I held up a copy of the EKG and lab tests.

"Son, since I am thirty years older than you, I wish I had your heart. It's perfectly fine and your pipes are wide open and unclogged."

He continued to jitter. "Are you sure, really sure?"

Just then, Bernard came strolling over from the desk where he was killing time and listening to this whole conversation. He gently reached over and pushed on the sore chest muscle.

"OW! Je-sus!" The kid jumped from the pain.

With the face of a wise sage delivering bad news, Bernard looked straight into the young soldier's eyes. "You either pulled a muscle or you've got a classic case of Updog Syndrome."

The now wide-eyed kid almost screamed, "What's Updog?"

Bernard calmly replied, "Nothin', dawg. What's up witch you?"

It took a couple of seconds for the joke to click, but as the soldier saw Bernard cackle his way back to the desk and me standing with a big grin, he realized we weren't bullshitting him about his heart. A mild tranquilizer for a night or two of nonfrightening sleep, and he would be fine.

In the background during all of this came a bunch of grunting and wheezing noises. Mike was putting the colonel through a thorough and grueling exam. That meant lots of rapid-fire bending, twisting, squatting, and lifting. Now that the exam was finished, all Mike thought the office commando needed was some ibuprofen and he would be fine. Obviously, that didn't sit well with the Vicodin-seeking brass-hole. So after talking to Mike, I decided I would give the colonel three little Vicodin, for nighttime use only. (We do not want to mask the pain, sir, and remember you need to be thinking clearly when you are doing all that paperwork.)

On his way out, the colonel and I almost collided as I was heading to check more X-rays.

"Say, Doc, I didn't mean to come off too hard on you there, you know what it's like when you're hurting. Tempers get a little short. Wondering if I could catch a favor from you, though."

Shit, he wanted more than three Vicodin.

"I've got some leave coming up. The pain pills might make me a little constipated plus me and the girlfriend are planning on meeting up back home for a little R and R, if you know what I mean . . ."

Home. We've got this wounded kid we want to get to back home and he sure isn't going for a little fun.

". . . and I was wondering if you could give me something to loosen me up . . . Plus maybe a few Viagras to make the weekened a little more, you know, action-packed."

Viagra? You think we have Viagra in the pharmacy in the middle of Iraq? Why in hell's name would we stock Viagra in a fucking war zone?

With a solemn look I answered, "Sorry, sir, I don't have everything you need for your trip but I do have something that might help get things moving. We don't carry any name brands but we do have a generic, it's called docusate. Take one in the morning and by nighttime, things will be functioning just fine. Guaranteed."

He winked at me. "Thanks, Doc. Let's make this our little secret, okay?"

I winked back. "Okay, sir. It's definitely a secret."

The real secret is that docusate is one of the most effective stool softeners known to medicine.

One of the medics interrupted my little vision of the colonel's toilet vacation. Time to head to the OR. Stat. When I got there, Rick and Bernard had already scrubbed in and were heading to the operating table. A quick-moving Rick looked back over his shoulder, "Dave, hustle and wash up. Kill the germs but don't stay for the funeral, we've got to move it."

A few cursory scrubs of the hands and I was in the room, watching the staff turn our kid onto his stomach so we could get at the back of his oozing neck. His face still looked young and at peace, but his vital signs told a different story. Blood pressure in the toilet. Rapid and irregular heartbeat. Hypothermic. Not only oozing from the neck, but now the leg, arm, and abdomen. A classic case of trauma shock. Irreversible. He would never leave the OR alive.

We usually boomed some Rolling Stones or Led Zeppelin when we worked, but today's OR was quiet. Just our low murmurs and the beeping of the monitors. The overheated OR caused steam to swallow us, fogging goggles and glasses, and filling our gloves with sweat. Looking up, we saw a crowd of noses pressed to the plastic windows of the door. By now, everyone in the hospital knew we had a young GI who was ready to die. I wondered how many knew he had a wife and two little kids.

My job was simple. Hold retractors and suction blood as fast as it flowed, opening a clear field of vision for Rick and Bernard to pull off some surgical miracle. And it would need to be a miracle. The leak was somewhere deep at the base of the skull, right next to the top vertebra. There had to be a small blood vessel in there with a microscopic tear. But even if we found it, there wasn't any way to tie it off—the space was so narrow, you couldn't fit a baby's finger in there, let alone that of an adult.

We spoke sparingly, all thinking the same thing. This kid was not going to die on us. Plain and simple. We had to get him home to see his family again. My mind added its own thought to theirs: this was not going to be like Columbine.

One hour turned into two, then three. I wondered, How was this kid hanging on? Bad question because as soon as the thought zipped through my brain, the rhythmic beep of the cardiac monitor went into the steady screech of cardiac arrest. We ripped the surgical drapes off, spun the kid over to get at his chest, and then hit him with the paddles.

One shock didn't do anything. Neither did the second. But the third was the charm. We had bought another chance.

Spinning him back, Rick and Bernard went on meticulously dissecting tissue away to try to find some angle to get at the leak. More hours passed. The noses stayed pressed to the windows. And we changed our gloves twice, spilling what seemed like buckets of sweat onto the floor. Blood continued its steady drip onto our boots. At a critical point when Bernard was carefully trying to work around a small nerve, the OR suddenly shook from the force of a rocket landing just outside the gate. The scalpel jerked against a nearby artery, slicing it in two, and sending a pulsating geyser of blood onto our masks and protective glasses. Temporarily blinded, we froze in fear, not daring to move with sharp instruments in our hands. Coolly, Bernard gently wiped clear a narrow window on his goggles with a sterile gauze while placing a finger on the jagged edges of the spurting vessel. His skills as a cardiac surgeon gave him the dexterity of a concert pianist; stabilizing the separated edges of the artery with one hand, he tied off the bleeding with the invisibly flying fingers of the other. A huge sigh of relief trapped itself inside my mask.

Five and a half hours and yet another cardiac arrest into the surgery, Bernard and Rick saw daylight. An artery smaller than the narrow lead of a mechanical pencil, almost completely hidden behind a piece of glistening white neck bone. Pulsing away lifeblood second by second, there was no way to clamp or tie off the leaking vessel. Then you could almost see the simultaneous light bulbs go on in Rick and Bernard. Bone wax. A few pennies' worth of cheaply manufactured material made from beeswax. The guys cautiously wedged in a small piece, then another, and the oozing gradually . . . slowly . . . stopped.

Blood pressure went up. Pulse rate slowed. Bingo.

"Let's get out of here real fast, guys," Rick whispered, as if the evil artery might hear him and start bleeding again.

It wasn't a home run, but at least the kid was still in the game. Realistically, the outlook was bleak. He had brain damage, some paralysis, and was still on life support. But at least we might be able to get him back to the States where some of the super-docs could do more than we could in our little tent hospital in the middle of the desert. Back home, his wife and loved ones had no idea of the miracle that Bernard and Rick had just performed.

We trudged together in the dark to midnight chow, no words between us, just the sand-filled wind in our faces. I thought about the three of us, strangers who by chance volunteered for the exact same deployment, were randomly placed in the same CSH in Iraq, and formed an unspoken brotherhood when we scrubbed in for our first case together. Tonight it all came together for the one case that needed a miracle. We had given it all we had . . . together.

At one minute after midnight we heard, then saw, the nightly plane to America. Our guy was on his way.

Rick finally broke the silence.

"You know why I didn't want to quit? The picture of his wife and kids. I don't know if you guys saw it, but every time I wanted to just let this guy go peacefully, I saw that picture."

Bernard broke in. "Man, you saw it, too? I thought we were

screwed. Then that picture kept on showing up in my head. It was a miracle we found that bleeder."

My smile was invisible in the dark.

With my mind on his family, as well as my own, I wondered aloud, "I just hope we did the right thing. You know, that it was worth it. I hope she's okay . . . and the kids, too."

Still thinking, I paused for a second. "I don't know. Maybe we went too far."

But we hadn't. At the same time that the plane from our CSH was taking off for home, a small group in America was getting ready for their own trip. The U.S. Army was flying the family of our wounded soldier to a hospital where they would see their husband and dad once more. We had succeeded in keeping him alive for an important, final family reunion. They now had a chance to say goodbye.

Several days later, they turned off his life support and the family donated his organs to others in need. And we suited back up into our mental armor, waiting to see who we would work on next.

DEAR KIDS

IT SEEMED LIKE I had already lived a lifetime of war in the course of a few short weeks. Though I tried to call home regularly, there often wasn't the time or desire to get into the details of life. Most often a call consisted of simply reassuring the person on the other end of the line that all was well. One evening after another eighteen-hour day, I finally had the time to drop an e-mail with a few extra details of life in Paradise.

From: david.w.hnida@us.army.centcom.mil
Sent: 06/22/07 23:08
To: hnidafamily2@aol.com

Hi Guys,

   We've got a little break in the action, so I thought I'd drop a quick note. Man, what a few weeks. We've got Internet in the phone tent right next to the ER so I can just run over and type a few syllables when we hit a lull. The computer crawls so slowly, I think it operates on hamsters

running on a little wheel—so this e-mail will probably take
an hour to write and send. Our phone/e-mail tent is not only
convenient, it's off limits to anyone but hospital personnel
and better yet, free.

*As I wrote the kids about the Internet, I thought about our first day
in camp when we were almost snookered into buying Internet for our
room. For a couple hundred bucks a month, we could sit in the luxury
of our quarters rather than wait in line. A couple of guys took the hook
and signed up—but it turned out their service is slower than the phone
tent and is always breaking down. The guys peddling the service are
pricks; it seems someone is always trying to make a quick buck during
a war and we docs rotating through must have a "Sucker" sign stuck to
our backs.*

*I went back to writing, trying to hurry before the next chopper de-
livered some business.*

But remember, all of our phone calls can be tapped and
our e-mails read, so there's a lot I can't say or write.

*In reality, there were bundles of things I wanted to tell them, but
there were simply too many thoughts, as well as things I simply didn't
want them to know.*

Things have been steady but not too crazy. I run a
trauma team in the ER and am the first doctor the patients
see when they are flown in.

*And I always pray I won't be the last face they will ever see. The
haunting thought keeps me up at night. My biggest fear is having an
overload of wounded come in, then having to pick the most critical and
decide to let him die because he'd take too much time and resources
from the others.*

The helipad is right outside the door of the ER—
maybe a hundred feet or so—when a chopper thunders in,
the whole camp shakes like a rag doll. The sensation starts
in your feet, then slowly works its way up to your teeth.
I've had a couple of landings where my mouth hurt from the
jarring vibrations of spinning blades. We don't need jeeps
or vehicles to bring patients to us, instead we use
large-wheeled stretchers called "rickshaws" which move as
fast as the medics can push them. I have to admit,
the injuries are a little different than what I'm used to back
home.

Like the guy who took some shrapnel to his eye, and when I tried to examine him the bloody jelly oozed down his cheeks and stuck to my gloves. Or the fellow who came in with a rib sticking out of his side—except it wasn't his rib. It belonged to the guy sitting next to him in the Humvee when it hit an IED. I still haven't slept through the night yet—too wound up to fall asleep or stay asleep for more than a few minutes if I finally do nod off. But at least I haven't puked since that first day. But I have lost about ten pounds in the past few weeks; it's called the "Scared Shitless in Iraq Diet."

The best way to describe where I work is to have you
flip on an episode of *M*A*S*H*—it's like a picture postcard.
Mainly tents, a couple of beat-up buildings, even some
containers, the kind you sometimes see on the back of big
tractor-trailers. Very claustrophobic, in fact our OR is half
tent, half container with very little room to move.

Surgerizing in close quarters made for some uncomfortable coziness. We often wore our pistols and as we pressed against each other, would quip about our discomfort.

"Is that your pistol, or are you just happy to see me?"

Or in the case of our resident stud, "Oh, sorry, Bernard. I meant, is that a shotgun or are you just happy to see me?"

Quarters were so tight, it wasn't unusual to have the weapon leave a bruise on our legs.

The ER is in one of the few actual buildings at the hospital. It's a little ramshackle but it's nice to have a solid roof over your head. Long and narrow with clanging metal doors at both ends, the wounded come in the front and are taken, the worst first, to the far end. Walk out the back door, hang a quick left, and you're at the OR tent.

Guys, you wouldn't believe this, but there is no door to the OR. Instead there's an old blanket that covers the entrance. When you sweep the blanket away and go in, you find yourself in a small tent. Straight ahead is OR number 1, to the right, OR number 2. Both small rooms are made from the containers with flimsy wooden doors separating the tent from containers. It seems like a fine, sandy dust creeps in through every ill-fitting opening and crack. People in the States would faint if they were ever brought to this makeshift surgical suite. So would the surgeons.

The Army Medical Corps calls our work "Damage Control Surgery." We had another name for it: spaghetti-and-meatball surgery—a unique brand of fast-food medicine. Simply put, our job was to keep the wounded soldier alive so someone in Germany or the States could do the compli-cated fancy repairs. There often wasn't time for us to do anything fancy. When a bullet or a bomb tears the human body apart, you might have fifteen minutes to isolate and stop the pulsating flow of blood from mul-tiple wounds. Take sixteen minutes and your patient dies. Someone's brother, sister, mother, or father is gone because you were one minute too slow. Our surgeries tend to be a sprint rather than a marathon.

I'm adjusting okay to life in the desert, just mainly trying
to get used to the heat. We hit anywhere from 120 to 135
degrees every day. But at least it's a dry heat. Then again
so is a microwave. We've also got this ever-present wind
whipping down from Turkey. We call it the "Tongue of Fire."
It blows at a steady, scorching 20 mph and we pray one
day it will just get tired and peter out. Whenever you walk
somewhere, it feels like someone is pointing a giant hair
drier right into your face.

*I don't think I've ever had my contacts stick to my eyes because of
heat, but that's what happened the other day. The whistling of the wind
is ghostlike and threatens to drive us insane. The best way to describe
it is like having a medical practice on the surface of the sun. If this is
a commercial for global warming I'm living in, we are all going to fry
one day.*

It's funny how we hustle from place to place. The
buildings and tents are air-conditioned and we trade speed
for heatstroke as we journey from one structure to the next.
The one place that can get steamy is the OR.

*In the States, operating rooms were kept chilly during routine sur-
geries to slow blood loss. In Iraq, it's the opposite—the air-conditioning gets turned down. The warm room helps prevent shock in a soldier
who has lost a lot of blood. We'd sweat so much our gloves would
fill to the point we could empty the liquid into a couple of coffee
cups.*

You'd love the crappers here, we have a bunch of porta-
johns scattered around the camp, but the best place to
drop a deuce is at what's called the "unisex" bathroom at

the hospital. Unisex means just that—it's for both males
and females . . . simultaneously if necessary. I remember
the first day I walked into the unisex. I was impressed—six
stalls, no waiting. But the true meaning of the word "unisex"
didn't sink in until I sat down and was suddenly surrounded
by female voices to the left of me, female voices to the
right—all accompanied by the sounds that come with sitting
on a toilet.

So far in this war, I'd pooped in a barrel, a small ravine, even a
sawed-in-half plastic bottle, but never in the presence of females. I
was so freaked, I would have shit my pants, except they were bunched
around my ankles. After the first few times, it's become like standing
and having a conversation with a neighbor over a picket fence. Talking
about the weather or how the tomatoes were growing.
"Hi, Dr. Hnida."
"Hi, ladies. And how are we today?"
"Fine. Sure looked pretty nasty this morning."
"Yup, but the sky is clearing."
"How's Colonel Reutlinger?"
"A little grouchy. You know, he gets a lot of aches and pains when
the weather changes. Then again, he can just be an ornery old coot."
"I've got some really nice salve from home that'll make his joints
feel good as new."
"Thanks much. I'll tell him to stop by. Have a good one."
"See you later, sir. Have a nice day, yourself."
Flush.

The nurses are great. Smart as can be, but soft and
tender to everyone that comes through. I've already learned
a lot from them. Sometimes I don't know how they deal with
the sadness that lies in the beds of our hospital.

*One of their stress relievers, I'd learned, was to light up. Every eve-
ning, a group of nurses would gather in some quiet place and puff away
on stogies while letting their stresses drain away. The first time I spied
the smoke rising from a meeting of the exclusive "Nurses Cigar Club"
I did a double take. I never realized women could puff away with the
skill, and look, of a bunch of bar-brawling tough guys.*

My quarters are pretty good—better than what I had
last time. It's an actual building instead of a tent, and I have
an actual bed instead of a rickety cot and sleeping bag.

*The dump called my room is actually palatial by combat zone stan-
dards. The first two floors of our three-story building were once open,
cavernous rooms, but add some ill-fitting plywood walls, and doors that
don't shut, and you've got housing. Most live two to a room with home-
made wooden bunk beds and creature comforts stuffed into every nook
and cranny. Not only are you squished, but the plywood is so thin you
can hear a symphony of snoring, farting, and groaning when you enter
the building at night.*

Some of the rooms have makeshift bunk beds to
squeeze out extra room, scary tall and scary rickety. One
of the ER docs, Gerry Maloney, fell out of the top bunk the
other night and scared the shit out of us. We thought a
rocket had scored a direct hit on the building.

*But those quarters are for the riffraff. Three of us lucked out and
got the Love Shack, the only room on the top floor, and with it a patio
complete with camouflage netting, sandbags to hide behind during a
gun battle, and stone floors that heat up to a little under 1,000 degrees
on a hot day. We've a bunch of pinups on the wall, put up by the original group of doctors to staff the hospital many moons ago. More super-*

stitious than sexist, we are paranoid to take the pictures down. Every day we say "good morning" to Ethel, Edith, Isabel, and the rest of the pinup crew, then add a good-luck pat to their bottoms before walking out to face the world.

My roommates are cool guys, one is a general surgeon, Ian Nunnally from Ohio, and a family doctor, Mike Barron from St. Louis. There's just the three of us rather than the twelve I lived with in 2004.

I lucked out with my roomies. We all work crazy hours so the key is keeping quiet day and night; it seems like someone is always trying to grab some shut-eye. Ian snores like a thunderstorm and likes a clean room; in fact he's such a neat guy I think he'd vacuum Iraq, sandy desert and all. Mike is quiet as a mouse, sometimes so quiet we've put a mirror under his nose when he is sleeping to make sure he's alive.

One small problem is my bed—because it is small. The Iraqis tend to be short and I don't fit very well at six-three on a metal bed frame made for the standard five-eight Iraqi. So I've stuffed a sleeping bag for padding over the metal railing at the end of the bed and let my legs hang off. I also have an easy chair, actually it's a folding chair with no back, but a full roll of duct tape was more than enough to make a solid surface to lean back on. It's such a piece of crap I think someone would actually have to pay someone to haul it away in a garage sale back home, but here it's a luxury item.

The doctors I work with are great guys, better than I could have hoped for. In fact, I don't think I've ever met a better group of doctors. We get along well. As Forrest Gump would say, we go together like peas and carrots.

My saviors, and those of my patients, came in the form of an odd mix of characters from across America. Seven other doctors who, like me, were reservists who volunteered to get the hell scared out of them. We are young and old; black and white; conservative and liberal.

My best friend is a surgeon from Oklahoma, a guy named Rick Reutlinger. We met the first day of the deployment and have been hanging out ever since.

It's said that opposites attract, and that certainly was the case with my battle buddy. I lucked out when Rick plopped his ample butt onto my lap for that bus ride to Fort Benning.

We eat together, exercise together, and perform surgery together. Like two grumpy old men, we spend most of our time yelling at each other, especially in the OR.

"Move your finger, Dave, or I'm going to lop it off! Where did you learn to play surgeon, anyway? Where did you get edumecated?"

"That's not my finger, asshead, it's his penis. Go back to that butcher's counter at the supermarket back home. They're asking for you."

Despite the yelling, there is never anger in the words. The man has a great bedside manner and truly the patience of a saint, especially when, showing my surgical inexperience, I would try to sew my glove to the patient we were trying to piece back together. ("Jesus, Dave, was you born with ten thumbs?")

Rick was a country-smart surgeon who knew his way around the human body better than any cutter I've ever met. He was named chief surgeon for good reason, and he's the main reason I haven't lost my mind yet.

Another close friend of mine is Bernard Harrison, he's a heart surgeon from Minnesota. We sometimes call him Harry.

You could do a pinup calendar of "The Doctors of Iraq" and could use Bernard for all twelve months. The women in the camp love him; so much so, there seems to be a constant stream of females knocking on his door at all hours. But he's never let one in; it seems he lives the life of a monk. We know that as a fact because we spy on him all the time.

He's also a helluva surgeon and is cool as ice. The guy became a camp legend last week when an Iraqi soldier shot in the chest came into the ER with the bullet lodged in his heart. He was a dead man until Harry cut open his chest right there in the ER, stuck a finger in the bullet hole, then calmly walked into the OR alongside the stretcher like the little Dutch boy with his finger plugging the hole in the dike. One keenly placed cardiac graft later and we had a young man who would hopefully live to a ripe old age.

But even legends have their share of rough cases, and they don't always have a Hollywood ending. Bernard was a top-notch cardiac surgeon in the real world and couldn't accept that in this world some wounds just aren't fixable. And even when you had a jaw-dropping performance, you still got shit on. After Bernard saved the Iraqi, he walked out of the OR and ran straight into one of the hospital administrators. Instead of "Holy shit" and "Great job," the first thing out of this guy's mouth was: "When do you think we'll be able to discharge him?" Discharge him? How about we just save him first, then make sure he doesn't die from surgical complications?

Stuff like that made the normally urbane Bernard's most widely used phrase a simple and profane one: "God, I hate this fucking war."

Our third surgeon is my roommate, Ian Nunnally. Great guy, especially to put up with me as a roommate. He comes from a military family and even served as an enlisted soldier himself before going on to medical school. An expert in burn care.

He's an enigma; how does an African American have such an Irish name? He explained it once but lost me somewhere over Great Britain. Kind of a libertarian by nature, it's not hard to guess his views on the war and society by the way he yells at the closed circuit TV every night. "Who the hell is running our country?" The question was sometimes followed by a well-thrown boot.

My other roommate, Mike Barron, is living proof of the old adage "You can take the man out of the Marines, but you can't take the Marine out of the man."

Mike's jarhead ways seem to have stuck with him, from the crew cut so flat you could set dinnerware on it to the ten-mile run he takes every day at the ungodly hour of 4 A.M. He never bitches about sleeping on a table in the middle of our room—hell, he never bitches about anything.

For a guy you would think would be the most hard-core, he seems the most liberal, always questioning why we can't go out on humanitarian missions to the villages and care for the Iraqi people. Flat head. Big heart.

Then there's Bill Stanton, he's our orthopedic surgeon. Considering how many people come through this place with messed-up bones, he is the busiest of all.

Bill simply doesn't have time for excruciating details. When I'd be stabilizing a new trauma arrival in the ER, he'd say, "Dude, just don't let him die. Find out what's broken, and then send him to the

OR. *I'll put him on my list." And when the dude got to the OR, Bill would be waiting with the song "Bad to the Bone" thumping out of his boombox.*

Unfortunately, I seem to make a specialty out of bugging the guy. Ortho is definitely not my best event, so I am either calling him for minor things or having him clean up my mistakes. But Wild Bill never gets pissed.

"Dude, you can sew that tendon. You don't need me. Here, let me show you, dude."

"Dude, you missed the tibia. I know you were getting hammered, but, dude, you gotta look at those films better."

For a forty-five-year-old West Point graduate, he sure likes the word "dude."

Our other ER doc is Gerry Maloney. Smart as hell, he's got this little '70s porn star mustache that I think is going to meet the razor one of these days. A little plump when we got here, he works out so much I bet he'll be a thin rail when we leave this place. He's as calm as a cucumber even when things get crazy busy.

Gerry has also got this high-pitched nasal monotone that would make a dog howl, plus he just loves military talk—and some other kind of talk none of us understands—like "that guy needs to run 40 into the wind." He leaves us bewildered whenever words exit his mouth. But we love him anyway and are lucky to have him.

The final member of the cast is our gas passer—Bob Blok aka Charlie Brown. Get it? Charlie Brown = Blockhead. A really funny guy, he is our anesthesiologist, and we appreciate the fact that he doesn't doze off or read magazines during long cases—afflictions that affect too many gas passers back home. Another good guy to have around.

The docs look out for each other pretty well, we each have our areas of expertise and weaknesses. But none of us feels shy about going and asking for help when we run into a jam. And none of us ever makes anyone feel stupid for asking a question, a radical difference from what I run into back home sometimes. In many ways it reminds me of when I was playing baseball—I never realized how much I miss having a group of best friends.

Kindness seems to be the middle name of the doctors I work with. More than once, I've collapsed in an exhausted heap after a long day or a tough surgery and awakened to find myself covered by a blanket that wasn't there when I feel asleep. And there's always a tray of food sitting waiting to be eaten since I've slept through a meal or two.

It's an interesting life here. We get up, go to breakfast, go to work, then come back to our rooms. Nowhere to drive to, no wheels to drive with. But then again, there's not much to see, we live in a small corner of the base and don't venture out. Our main way to blow off steam is to go to the gym and work out, which is something I do pretty much every day.

That's not to say there isn't entertainment if you want some. We doctors tend to stay on the sidelines but do get a front-row seat to the shenanigans that keep people sane during war. We don't booze it at all—it's not like M*A*S*H, where you knock down a couple of home-made martinis after a day of mayhem. We are on call 24/7 and always need enough warm bodies in case of incoming wounded. That's not to say the rest of the hospital lives the life of puritans. Anything but. If you want booze, it's available—much of it gin or vodka with blue food coloring and sent in mouthwash bottles, or small bottles of hooch stuffed in the cardboard rolls of toilet paper sent from home. Everyone knows *we need toilet paper here so no one thinks twice about inspecting boxes from home filled to the brim with TP. As for other substances, let's say I don't even want to know what comes out of the hookah that was smoked at parties.*

And if you wanted sex, you didn't need to go far. Some deeds were done in dark places—on top of the latrine, next to the laundry facility, your room if your roommate was gone (or even wasn't gone, feigning sleep). The best show in Iraq took place one night when a chopper circled round and round over the roof of the ICU for ten minutes with its bright spotlight shining on a couple coupling. God it was loud. Even the helicopter.

The best deal of all is if you were lucky enough to have a single room. One guy and his favorite nurse had a regularly scheduled afternoon delight in his private abode every day at 4 P.M. For a dollar a minute, we'd let soldiers borrow a stethoscope and listen through the plywood walls.

We do have some parties here; the week we arrived, we had a welcome shindig on the roof of our building complete with a live band from the 25th Infantry. Last week we had a toga party on the rooftop right outside my room.

Most of us wore our shorts under our sheets, but some wore nothing but the sheet, which made it easier to sneak off to dark corners for a quickie. It's funny, the invitees to these parties are mainly the worker bees from the hospital, I don't think the administrators are invited. The parties are held on a regular basis to maintain sanity. Up next: Elvis has left Iraq. I wish I were Elvis. I think we all wish we were Elvis.

I've got more but the tent and my teeth are starting to shake—a chopper is paying a visit, so got to run. Will call later. Love, Dad.

10

REBELS WITH A CAUSE

W E DECIDED THE day would be a good one. It was the Fourth of July and we were going to make sure America's birthday was celebrated in proper fashion. Except for the fact that as red-blooded American boys, we didn't want to see any red blood on this holiday.

The day started like most, with me bounding down the stairs to pick up Rick for a quick bite before rounds, pounding on the door, then launching into our daily repetition:

"A-B-C-D."

It seemed like I lived in a preschool world, from memorizing my alphabet to take care of patients, to listening to decades-old advice from my father, to reciting the letters with Rick before we launched off on some journey around the camp. I'd stand in Rick's doorway and we'd both go through reminders of essential equipment before we set out the door. Forget an item, and it was trouble.

"A" stood for arms; you always needed your pistol, even if you were just going for a run. "B" was for beeper, you carried your pager 24/7. "C" was for card, as in ID card. You couldn't get into any building without showing an official picture of your face, even if the guards knew you. And "D" stood for reflector belt. Or in Rick's terminology, deflector belt. Hence the "D." No sense arguing with his mangled logic.

The pistol was obviously important in a war zone, but when we wore it in a holster when dressed in exercise shorts and official Army T-shirts, there was no place to put the clips of ammunition. So we'd just leave our bullets behind, figuring we could always just throw our pistols at the enemy if the camp was attacked. After all, it was the administrators' bright idea for us to leave our helmets and body armor at the hospital for safekeeping; I guess they felt confident the insurgents would be courteous and wait for us to sprint down and get our stuff before they started shooting or mortaring us.

The deflector belt was probably the least essential of all. It was a simple elastic belt with a band of reflective material around it so the wearer could be seen at night. A good concept, except perhaps in a war zone where bad people with sniper rifles tend to lurk. But the omnipotent hospital administrators made their views clear: "We'd rather you get shot than run over by a truck." So you got yelled at if you went out—day or night—without your reflector belt escort. I guess it was a matter of playing the odds.

Otherwise, our life was like the movie *Groundhog Day*. Each day a repeat of the day before, and the days before that. We'd stumble over to a hasty breakfast, tell a few jokes, and stare bleary-eyed at a babbling TV. Like most days at Paradise General, we had no idea of what we were in for, an uncertainty that was hard on all of us. Its price was restless sleep—that's if sleep would even come—and a never-ending search for distractions, whether it be hours spent jogging in the predawn heat or counting the porta-potties on the base. Our shared misery also found solace in the uniquely male world of ballbusting.

The initial July 4th target was anesthesia. The tussle sounded just like the civil wars in hospitals back home: "In this corner, trying to put people to sleep while staying awake themselves: anesthesia. And in the far corner, a masked man with a sharp knife and giant ego: the surgeon. Let's get ready to rummmmm . . . ble."

It was no different here; surgeons and gas passers took special pleasure slicing each other with insults.

"Colonel Blok, what's the deal with your patients? They keep on waking up when I'm trying to cut on them. Jeez, you couldn't put a guy with narcolepsy to sleep."

"Reutlinger, even if you had the world's sharpest scalpel you couldn't cut a good fart."

Next on the fight card; surgeon pitted against surgeon.

"Harry, you know Captain Dee was asking about you," Rick said.

"That's right, Bernard, she was slinking around looking for your room last night. Making believe she was lost," I added.

Shaking his head rapidly and feigning indignation, Bernard answered, "What's with you guys? She doesn't like me. And I've got no time for any of this tomfoolery. Sweet Jesus, get back to your oatmeal."

Rick looked at me across the coffee-stained white tablecloth.

"I don't know any Tom Foolery. And Sweet Jesus isn't going to help you if she sinks her claws into you."

Back home, we wouldn't have thought of doing it, but in our world of war-induced immaturity, out it came: "Harry and Captain Dee sitting in a tree. K-I-S-S-I-N-G. First comes love, and then comes marriage, then little Harry in a baby carriage."

Bernard sputtered, then snorted a laugh.

"You guys are useless. I'm third call today, so don't bother me unless someone needs a bypass. I'm heading to work out."

Bernard was easily the camp Adonis. It seemed like every unattached woman, and probably a few married ones, swooned when he walked into a room. He was, by nature, sweet and smooth, but did little to encourage their flirtations and advances. Yet still they came, whether it was to the OR, the ER, the gym, or his room. Especially his room. So often, we thought it might be a good idea to put up one of those little "take-a-number" machines, the same kind you see at the supermarket deli, at the end of the hallway.

"*Number 22. Now serving number 22 for Lieutenant Colonel Harrison. Ma'am, what would you like today?*"

"*I'll take 195 pounds of that gorgeous hunk, please.*"

Man, we could have made a lot of money being pimps for this guy.

After rounds, I trotted through every building and tent of the hospital, searching for the perfect cup of coffee, something thick, black, and possessing the ability to dissolve a spoon. I was on an anti—foofoo crusade. Then it was time to head to the ER and juggle paperwork with patients.

A few weeks earlier Colonel Quick had handed out job titles; while Rick was named chief surgeon, I drew the official title of "Chief of Quality Assurance," which meant I had to oversee and review everyone's work. In my mind, my real title was "King of the Hospital." The staff celebrated the coronation by making me a cardboard crown, and giving me a celebratory parade around the hospital in a wheelchair throne while I knighted a few folks with the touch of a crutch. I especially loved hearing "Your Royal Highness" as I rode, though the doctors tended to address me as "Your Royal Anus."

In truth, there was little to oversee—everyone did high-quality work—and all I needed to do was simply scribble my glowing monthly report.

When I got to the ER, there was Rick, hiding out trying to avoid hemorrhoid patients in sick call. As I walked in empty-handed of real coffee and resigned to a not-so-perfect cup of Cinnamon Surprise, I heard a new round of ballbusting.

"Nice head, sir."

"Need to borrow some floor wax to brighten that shine?"

"They're asking for you over at the pool hall, sir. Seems the cue ball is missing."

Rick had just gotten a super-buzz-cut haircut the day before, and now was a bright shining beacon for the medics' jokes. They all wore sunglasses to cut down the glare from Rick's head.

"Dr. Reutlinger, I think there's a blown-up condom sticking out of your neck."

He was always a good sport, even though the ones flinging the insults were young enough to be his kids.

In fact, it was a special treat for all of us when Rick came wandering through the workplace—it was as if he wore a sign on his back that said, "Please Poke Fun at Me."

That meant a not-too-ill patient who needed a surgical consultation often got a pompous introduction: "I'm going to have a specialist come in and examine you. He's right over there. Rick Reutlinger, MD—Mentally Deranged."

Or a whispered warning to an unsuspecting patient.

"Ever hear that bad things tend to happen in threes? Well, Dr. Reutlinger has already killed his three patients this week, you're number four so you're safe. But first let him go outside and have a drink to steady his hands."

Rick would just roll his eyes and say a two-syllable Oklahoma-twanged, "Da-ve."

Maybe that's why we all got along so well—it was no harm, no foul. We'd slam each other, the staff would slam us, and no one got offended or acted like an arrogant asshole.

In honor of the holiday, a few of the female medics stuffed socks into their crotches for the "extra built" look. I decided I would wear an oversized "Uncle Sam" hat while working. And asked which doctor I was going to be for the day. The medics started scribbling on strips of adhesive that I'd tape to my shirt. The choices were many: Dr. Lance Boyle, Dr. C. Menn, and Dr. Jacques Strapp. The winner was a play on a common bumper sticker seen on the back of some tractor-trailers: "How's my doctoring? Call 1-800-TOUGH-SHIT."

Rick shook his lightbulbed head in mock despair.

"You're going to get in big trouble one of these days, Davy-boy."

Yet Rick couldn't claim total innocence in our world of pranks.

It was his idea when we were finished using the porta-potty to put up a sign that said, "Mission Accomplished."

And his idea to speak fake Japanese to the chow hall workers or other camp staff every Monday while making Tuesday fake Norwegian day. He even invented a new language—"Charabic," a combination of Chinese and Arabic. We had no idea how to speak either language; then again, Rick couldn't speak decipherable English.

And it was his idea to develop a different style of walking for our daily treks to the hospital. His favorite was Wednesday, the day we "walked like an Egyptian" across the camp.

But not everyone had a healthy sense of humor. Especially some of the administrators, a group whom some of the medics referred to as the "Three Stooges." Moe, Larry, and Curly just walked by the doctors as if we were invisible—and that was courteous treatment compared to what they offered the hospital staff. Worse, the pompous trio would often stroll around the ER with their pistols strapped on while we were dealing with a roomful of patients. For some reason they thought they were immune from the "all weapons must be locked up" rule. The medics would quip, "That guy thinks he's Dirty Harry or something." I dreamed of the day one of them was going to shoot himself by accident and I would say, "Sorry, I'm not a proctologist so I don't know how to take care of someone like you."

The Army pissed us off, too. There was one case in particular that boiled our eggs—a day Rick had worked for hours trying to save a kid with a bad belly wound. The case was a messy one and by the time Rick finished, he could literally wring his socks of the blood that had spilled off the body and run down his legs. Since all the squeezing in the world couldn't save those socks, they went straight into the trash, and Rick went off to meet me at chow. That's where he was turned away: no socks, no service. And no explanation in the world could grant him a reprieve and a meal. Even: *I'm a surgeon—long case—critical patient—lots of blood—you don't want that blood in here—you stop serving in five minutes—no time to go to the barracks and get a fresh pair.*

Sorry, sir. Next time you'll plan ahead.

Right, and next time we'll tell the blown-up soldier to plan ahead.

Maybe that's why Bill wears big rubber fireman boots into his cases—the blood simply runs off like rainwater.

At times, a special stone in our boots was the active duty guys, a few of whom regarded us as kids with cooties on their schoolyard. Being a reservist was bad enough for some of the active duty elite— but being a *reservist doctor* was the equivalent of the military homeless. Holding signs on the corner of the hospital: *"Will operate for food."*

They were spit-and-polish, we were just . . . spit. And blood. I guess the bottom line for them was reservists weren't "real soldiers," and doctors, well, we weren't even "fake soldiers," an insult made worse by the fact most of us were handed the rank of major or lieutenant colonel simply by joining their army.

It wasn't all of the active duty folks who turned their noses at us; we actually got along with and genuinely liked most of the men and women who made the military their career. And vice versa. It was simply a small group, the *Lord of the Rings, Iraq Edition* fobbits that gave us the hardest of times. And on our base, we were overrun with fobbits.

Though I needed a translator for most Army-speak, even I understood the term given to those who never left the safety of a base in a war zone. Most of our camps were designated as a Forward Operating Base—or a FOB. Their home-bound occupants were therefore christened "fobbits." The fobbits would usually spend their deployments never seeing or interacting with an honest-to-goodness Iraqi. And when you did the math, fobbits made up close to the majority of soldiers stationed in Iraq. They might just as well have picked a different desert for all the Iraqis they saw.

Tucked away in safe corners, or really the safe innards, of a large

base, these soldiers just got up every day, walked to work at some office or shop, and never went outside the wire. It was like going to work
back home in the States, not that their sacrifices weren't substantial;
after all, they were apart from their loved ones for twelve to fifteen
months at a time. And that sucked. But when a small number of them
shit on us, that sucked even more, especially for those of us who did
get to see real Iraqis every day, usually bleeding ones.

We had a small and special group of fobbits who were our designated tormentors—sort of like schoolyard bullies, or in this case,
more like pains in the ass since we usually outranked them. They
would confront us in the mess hall with accusations of a sloppy uniform: *Sir, your pants aren't tucked into your boots properly and your
shoelaces aren't tucked into your boots.* Or would admonish us for sitting with our enlisted coworkers: *Sirs, no fraternization allowed. You
need to set a good example for the other troops.* We'd just shake our
heads and walk away.

One day the fobbits went too far. An exhausted Ian had just finished a marathon surgery, changed out of a bloody uniform into his
workout clothes, and headed to chow. As he stood in line, a group of
sergeants surrounded him, saying his shorts and T-shirt weren't regulation, and that he should leave the mess hall. After he told them to
screw off and sat down with steam coming out of his ears, we could
see the fobbits sitting at their table pointing and laughing at us. We
decided to pay them a quick house call on our way out.

"Gentlemen, we have sharp knives to cut your skin, thick tubes to
stick up your dicks, and rigid tubes to shove up your asses. Sometimes
we confuse what goes where. You ever talk to us again—even look at
us again, we'll experiment with our tools until we get it right. Now
your meals are over. Get up. Get out. And say, 'Yes, Sir,' as you leave."

They never bothered us again.

It was tougher when we had to deal with those who outranked
us—so we could only make fun of them behind their backs. Like
General Richard Head. He was the general you've probably never

heard of, but General Richard Head was actually a pretty important guy in this war. A generic make-believe leader for those of us who actually got our hands dirty every day. We loved him so much we even referred to General Head by his nickname, Dick. If we ever had a bitch, moan, or complaint, it was always nice to have a General Dick Head to blame it on.

Don't get me wrong, the Army had some great leaders we trusted and respected. I actually liked a lot of our generals. And rumor had it, a couple even thought I was okay as well, even though during my first deployment they seemed to take great pleasure in chewing big chunks out of my ass. But the man who wore the star wasn't always what he seemed to be, especially when his personal photographers were around.

Take the one general who the medics told me wanted to give some medals and commemorative coins to our brave troops wounded in battle. The problem was, at the time, we had no brave troops wounded in battle. Our beds were empty of wounded soldiers; they'd either been fixed or shipped off to Germany. The only American in the ward was moaning and groaning from a recent surgery. The general didn't care, he was going to give this suffering soldier a commemorative coin. Unfortunately, when he found out the poor kid was in pain from hemorrhoid surgery, the general wanted his coin back. Hemorrhoid Man wasn't going to give it up without a fight, pain in the ass or no pain in the ass. The tug-of-war must have looked great on camera.

Then there was the guy with stars in his eyes and on his shoulders who came to visit our hospital for his own photo op. We were ordered to dress nice, look sharp, and stay put in the ER. Under any circumstances, DO NOT LEAVE, you never know when he'll walk in. But after an hour of a painfully boring wait for an overdue general, my bowels decided they could wait no longer. So I headed to the latrine. And finished up my business just in time to bump into the general as *he* rushed in to use the facilities. I offered him my newspaper but all I got was a scowl in return, along with a dressing-down from an administrator as I walked out of the latrine. It was the first time I've been yelled at for pooping since I was three years old.

The pranks and jokes and funny stories made up a potent prescription for sanity in the land of carnage. We hoped our self-prescribed Rx would especially be helpful on our nation's birthday. In many ways it was, but it wasn't enough.

When the first radio call came in, the Uncle Sam hat was flung aside, the nametags ripped off, and socks pulled out of crotches. The wrong kinds of fireworks were detonated that day, and the wounded came in wave after wave. It was one of our worst days, but it was hard to feel sorry for ourselves. The day would always be remembered by the wounded as *their* worst day; our job was to see them through it.

When the birds ceased their deliveries, the staff all seemed to wear vacant eyes, slack jaws, and slumping shoulders. The room displayed its own decorations: a floor slickened by blood, the litter of discarded bandages, and a mix of shredded and blackened clothes that once were the property of our guests.

It was not a happy Fourth of July.

11

ANATOMY OF A TRAUMA

IJUST LAY IN my bunk staring up at the metal support where my wristwatch hung. A not-so-glamorous Timex sports watch—I had worn this one for more than four years, and at the bargain price of thirty bucks, I'd more than gotten my money's worth. It's got a lot of timers, calculators, and stopwatches—though all I used were the basic "what time is it" function and the alarm. Not that I even needed the alarm on days I was scheduled to pull a day shift, as I always woke up early and thought about the great unknown called the ER and what surprises would be delivered by air.

It was only 5:15 when my eyes came to life—the alarm wasn't set to buzz for another hour and my work shift didn't start until 7:00. I rolled over and saw Mike was already up and out—for his daily run in the cool darkness of the morning. In this part of the country, that meant a chilly 90 degrees.

Next to my watch, I kept pictures of my family. It was only 3:15 in the afternoon *yesterday* for them—and I hoped they were having a decent day; I had no idea what mine would be like. Some days were quiet, others chaotic; but the war didn't publish a schedule of the wounds that will be suffered on a particular day, and it was the not knowing that made me crazy. When I sat at my makeshift desk in the ER, I could never fully relax; it was a twelve-hour fidgeting exhibition that kept me from reading or watching a movie with the medics if business was slow.

I started every morning with a quick prayer that I would do a good job, and most importantly, that I wouldn't hurt anyone. I'd mumble the same prayer back home before going to work every day. A little bit of the Bible came next. I usually read from something called "The Message"—a version of the Good Book without all of the "thee's" and "thou's"; instead it was filled with simple language such as "Jesus told the moneychangers to take a hike." That kind of religious talk I could understand.

Just as there are no atheists in foxholes, I doubted there were many in combat hospitals. Not that I experienced a sudden conversion when I got here; I spent a few minutes every morning back home reading and contemplating, as well as regularly asking God to cut me some slack for not always being His most faithful servant.

Bill told me he had found a nice, easygoing Catholic mass up at the 82nd Airborne, and each week he'd asked if I'd like to tag along. I should. But since joining the Army, organized religious services and I haven't gotten along very well. Seems like there's a lot of Holy Roller stuff, and I didn't do well with praying for God to gird my loins as a warrior. Military-style "Hooah church" gave me spiritual indigestion. Yet I hadn't been thrown into some deep morass of asking God why he allowed all this bloodshed, even with all of the gore we've had to wade into. After all, it wasn't anything new—mankind has been slaughtering each other since the Stone Age when we crushed each other over the head with rocks and clubs. Except now, the rocks explode and the clubs shoot bullets. Nice to see how much we've evolved and become civilized; at times, I wondered if this war would ever end. No matter, Bill's discovery sounded like a religious gold mine yet I still hadn't gone for an injection of spirituality. I would simply continue to pray I didn't hurt anyone.

By the time my morning musings had ended, the clock had fast-forwarded to 0615. I shook out my uniform and boots free of any scorpions or spiders, grabbed my pistol, and headed down to pick up Rick.

He, too, had been up for hours. We didn't talk much about our stresses, but I knew the pressure of being chief surgeon had cut into his sleep and ability to relax.

It was my day to run the ER; Rick was my on-call surgeon yet we didn't have to remind each other—the message of anxiety was clear in our eyes. We had only known each other for a little more than a month, yet we were already at a point where we could read each other's thoughts without uttering a word. We flew through our ABCs, made sure we had our gear, and then headed over for a meal of powdered eggs, which we simply pushed around on our plates. It seemed like we both knew we were in for it—how we knew I couldn't say—there was just a vibe that surrounded us. Even the usual jokes were missing in action as we made the trek from the chow hall to the hospital.

As I pushed open the ER doors, I mumbled a quiet "See you later." His answer was a terse "I know."

I greeted my medics with a quick "How is it going, folks?"

They replied in unison.

"Fine, sir, just another day in fucking paradise."

"That it is, my young friends. Say, I think I'm going to head over to rounds for a few minutes, page me if there's any business."

As I walked, I thought about our peculiar brand of work; it was unlike anything any of us imagined. The meat and potatoes of our daily life was trauma, but not like the stuff back home. There, it's a lot of blunt injury from car accidents with an occasional hole from a bullet or blade. Here our life was pulling nails from a car bomb out of someone's back. Amputating limbs hanging by a thread of skin. Trying to keep some guy's intestines from spilling onto the floor as you struggled to examine him. Comforting a young soldier who can't stop stuttering after seeing his best friend's brains splashed throughout the inside of a Humvee.

It could be mentally chaotic, but wasn't the emergency medicine you'd typically see on TV with yelling, screaming, and bedlam. I learned on that horrible first day in the ER that I needed calm. So the dual rules of my desert trauma center were simple, especially for visitors who stood in the peanut gallery: Keep quiet. And stay out of my way. I had lost my medical virginity on that inaugural day when my head went spinning. It was a day that now seemed centuries old. I had changed in ways I probably wouldn't discover until many years and miles passed between me and this hellhole.

I sneaked into the back of rounds and looked at my friends. Rick, Bernard, Bill, Mike, Gerry, Ian, and Blockhead—I rolled a lucky seven when I was put with these guys. They were good at their jobs, they were good to the patients, and they were good to the staff. And they were good to me—all at one time or another holding me by the hand when I was stumbling.

We all brought some piece of medical knowledge to the table, and were always willing to bail out someone who was drowning in a roiling sea of blood. At times, the group had been stunned into silence by the bodies or pieces of bodies brought to us on stretchers, yet none lost our patience or humanity. I saw my colleagues naturally laying a soft hand to the head of a scared, wounded soldier. They would kneel on one knee and gently talk the language of reassurance and confidence into the ear of the injured. And sometimes walk away with deep red indentations of the skin—a place where the frightened had latched on and painfully squeezed tight the arm of the doctor promising to aid them.

I was blessed with an orthopedist I could call out of bed in the middle of the night to look at an X-ray I didn't know how to read, and I worked with surgeons who never got angry when I lagged behind their rapid pace in the OR. I also learned it was not only me who had a good fairy who left food when I missed a meal, or a blanket when

exhaustion struck; we all looked out for the one who needed rejuve-
nation. We trusted each other with our lives, as well as the lives of the
soldiers we cared for.

Rick was in the corner with his eyes pointed at the floor, brow
furrowed and stressed. Not paying one damn bit of attention to what
was being discussed by the group. Sweat like ice water ran down my
neck—something was up. I decided I had better head back to the
ER and wait for the other boot to drop. It took less than two hours of
nervous toe tapping and three cups of foo-foo coffee before the morning's call came in.

And this is how it went:

09:11:30 I'm asking Major Boutin why in hell we are drinking
Blueberry Surprise instead of real coffee. The medics are telling dirty
jokes. Sergeant Courage is outside sweeping the sidewalk.

09:12:00 The radio crackles. A firefight has taken place after an
IED attack. Estimate two urgent casualties—arrival by helicopter
in twenty-five minutes. Condition unknown—so we prepare for four
patients and arrival in ten minutes. Information is often muddled
when called in from a thundering helicopter. The message sets in
motion a frantic cascade of rushing feet, hurried voices, and upset
stomachs.

09:12:30 I ask for pages to be put out to surgeons, orthopedics,
anesthesia, respiratory therapy, and X-ray. Maybe an extra ER doc or
two. We're going to need help with this one.

09:13:00 Staff heads to trauma bays—equipment is checked and
double-checked. Suction, defibrillators, emergency drugs. IVs are
hung and ready to drip. Chest tubes and intubation equipment placed
within reach. I double-check my personal gear: stethoscope, safety
glasses, and a pair of gloves. Then stuff more gloves into my pockets

in case things are extra bloody. I end the ritual with a quick pat-down of my shirt pockets for my emergency cheat cards. Haven't used them yet but the day I don't have them is the day I will need them.

09:14:00 We go in sets to the unisex latrine. Always have an empty bladder, you never know when you'll get the chance to go. As I stand emptying my bladder, the nurse in the stall next to me asks how my family is. *Just fine, thanks. Yours?*

09:16:00 Back in the ER, we share packs of specially designated "trauma gum"—Trident or Wrigley's to keep from getting cotton mouth. We walk, pace, and tell weak jokes. I have a crucifix in my left pocket that has been rubbed raw over the months during these walks. I pace seven steps toward the front door, then back for seven more. We all have our pre-trauma quirks—this is mine. Why seven? Mickey Mantle and John Elway wore No. 7. It has to be good luck.

09:19:00 Like Radar O'Reilly, we sense the vibrating blades of incoming medevacs before we hear them. They are eighteen minutes early. Medics go to the helipad wearing Mickey Mouse—eared hearing protection. The rest of us line up in our positions. I am at the head of the stretcher in Alpha bay waiting for the most critical case. I stand on the left—anesthesia on my right. Everyone in their assigned position. *It's like a football game. Just waiting to say "Hike."*

09:20:30 Medics come into the ER. Moving fast, not a good sign. Someone shouts: "Three urgents on litters." Sprinting medics rush in three soldiers. I eyeball the wounded from a distance . . . as well as the faces of the medics. Their stress tells me how worried I should be. *Shit, they look as old as I feel.* I hear moaning, see blood, and sense death. The worst of the three is blood-soaked and blue in color, he's missing part of a leg and has bright white bone fragments sticking out from his arm—the fragments are pointing oddly at the ceiling.

<u>09:20:45</u> I am multitasking, again eyeballing the wounded, listening to the flight medic reel off the wounds, blood pressures, and what happened in the field. Medics take the three to appropriate bays. I still have little idea what's wrong with my guy from my cursory look. *Focus, man, focus.* I shake off a shiver and my mind goes into a well-rehearsed auto mode.

<u>09:21:00</u> Like a preschooler, I recite my ABCs aloud: Airway, Breathing, Circulation. Then you worry about the other stuff. My guy fails "A"—he's not breathing. Check the airway—can't hear breath sounds when I put my stethoscope to his chest. The breathing tube is in the wrong place—his food pipe, not his lungs. It must have been chaos on the copter. I tell Dean Losee, the nurse anesthetist, to pull it and put in another. The medics are sticking in large IVs—can't do much until you've got a way to run in fluids and drugs. I see blood dripping on the floor from a place where a leg should be. Tourniquet is on—it's still not enough. *Man, this guy has a thick thigh—need to put on another tourniquet and make it tight!* Blood pressure 74/46, pulse 166. *Bad.* Clothing is cut off within ten seconds.

<u>09:21:30</u> Dean is struggling with the new tube for good reason—the patient's jaw is in pieces. I reach in and pull out blown-out teeth with a gloved finger while a medic suctions blood. It's the hardest tube Dean has ever done—he nails it on the first shot as I hold the Adam's apple and facial bones steady. Listen to lungs—*good air, Dean, good job.* We've got two big IVs—*good job medics*—but I need a bigger line since one arm is mangled.

<u>09:22:00</u> Call Rick into bay. He starts a central IV in a neck vein that leads directly to the heart. I have to ignore the missing leg and mangled arm—both have stopped dripping. Don't get distracted. They can wait. Need to look for smaller, innocent holes that snuck in deep and hit something bad.

<u>09:22:30</u> Back to the big picture—we've got IV access. Airway. Blood pressure still in the toilet. Heart rate still fast. Neck brace on. Need to continue exam. Abdomen is tight—probably bleeding internally. Pelvis feels loose. The bones grate and grind as I push and squeeze. *Damn! These bleed fast and will kill him before anything else.* Call for a binder to stabilize the pelvis—but sometimes the binders make certain types of fractures bleed more. I look to Ian for an opinion—he nods a go-ahead.

<u>09:23:00</u> We hustle X-ray in to take some pictures with their portable machine on wheels. Takes six of us to roll the patient—can't wait for the X-ray to put on binder—fingers crossed. While rolling patient—examine spine. Feel for ridges or drop-offs. Put a gloved finger in rectum—there's blood—so there's bleeding inside the pelvis or abdomen. *Not good.* As we turn the patient back, his blood pressure drops to 46/28 and pulse shoots to 180. *Did I make a mistake here?* I am now cornered by two rules of combat medicine: you cannot call time-out when things go bad, and there are no do-overs.

<u>09:24:00</u> Blood pressure up to 88/62. Pulse now 132. Some progress. Binder helped. Finish exam and call findings to trauma nurse. The soldier's injuries read like a textbook of trauma medicine: shock with dropping blood pressure and racing pulse, the rigid abdomen of internal bleeding, a shrapnel-peppered face and burns that have peeled away skin from his hands and legs. He's missing chunks of flesh. Bruising over left thigh? Fracture. *Billy will need to fix this as well.* I peek into the other bays and check on what's happening—other docs have things under control. Thank God for Gerry and Mike.

<u>09:25:00</u> One of the medics suctions the blood pouring from the soldier's mouth while I stick a finger back in—gloves swimming in blood as I try to discover its source. My index finger falls into a deep crevice where the gum used to be; gauze packing staunches the

bleeding. Blood pressure continues a steady ascent while pulse slows. I didn't make a mistake after all. The binder, tight tourniquets, and a few units of blood keep this kid in the race.

09:26:00 Patient starting to move—need more drugs to keep him out because of the breathing tube. I have no idea how bad his head injuries are—I didn't feel anything when I felt behind his head but I know his facial bones are a mess. Can't check pupils.

09:26:30 Billy checks arms and legs after my exam to get an idea of what is an emergency and what is not. The pelvis is fractured— the binder worked. Ian does a FAST exam—it's an acronym for Focused Assessment with Sonography in Trauma—basically a quick ultrasound of the abdomen to look for pockets of blood but he already knows this kid needs surgery—fast. I've gone through three pairs of gloves. Need to cut away all bandages placed in the battlefield—they weren't soaked so we had time. Now we'll look at the small potatoes of wounds.

09:27:30 Doctors all talk—who needs what—who goes first to the CAT scanner—how about the OR? My guy needs to be opened to check for internal bleeding. We've run in three units of O positive blood as well as other IVs already but blood pressure still down and pulse still up. Nurses notify OR we are coming fast. There may be shrapnel in the brain but it doesn't matter at this point—no time to check. Scan later—got to do some Hail Mary surgery and stop the internal bleeding—his brain won't matter if we don't get blood flowing to it.

09:28:00 I'm reassessing everything again—to make sure I didn't miss anything. I ask the head nurse what I've forgotten. She tells me we are good to go. The medics have already administered antibiotics and other drugs—we've worked quickly with nods of the head and a murmured "Yes" or "No." There's a peanut gallery watching the action but they stay out of the way and it's still fairly calm and quiet.

09:29:30 My guy is wheeled to the OR. Ian and Rick to work on him. Bernard has his hands full with the other two patients. Billy will follow up and work on bones once the damage control surgery is done. Blood pressure and pulse better but still making us nervous.

09:31:00 I call the CSH in Balad—the one with a surgeon who can fix facial bones—and tell him we've got a customer after our surgeons are done exploring the abdomen and ortho stabilizes the fractured pelvis and thighbone. We'll scan the head before we send and hope there's no shrapnel in it. Other patients go to X-ray and the CAT scanner—they are stable and will wait their turn for Bernard in the OR. I sign forms that authorize giving unmatched blood, a signature that would be medical malpractice back in the States.

I LOOK AT the second hand as it sweeps around the face of the clock on the dull green wall.

It took nine minutes from front door to OR for my patient. Nine minutes where I became a short story in this soldier's life. I realized he probably wouldn't remember me and we would never meet again.

Our surgeons fixed his internal injuries—including putting a lifesaving clamp on his large bleeding vessel. A CAT scan after surgery had good news: no shrapnel in the brain. He was stable enough to fly to Balad to have his face repaired, then on to Germany for further surgery. Then home.

By this time in our rotation, cases like this were taking on the feel of routine. Businesslike with a sprinkling of adrenaline-filled panic thrown in for flavor. I was drained but once again thankful for the medics and nurses who mentally pushed me to get the job done. They were my heroes. And heroes to the soldiers they saved.

We had no time to wring the sweat from our uniforms—another bird flew in about an hour later—no warning—it just dropped from the sky with more wounded. Our medics had just wrung out their blood-soaked mops from swabbing the floor when we heard the incoming blades beating the air. The day had just begun.

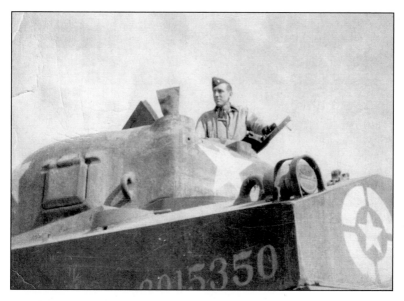

My dad, age 23, stationed in Italy, 1943.

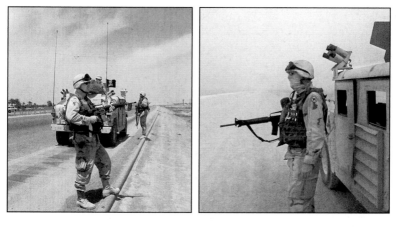

Armed with a rifle and medical supplies, I scan a field for insurgents outside
Baghdad.

2004: Stuck in a sandstorm on some
unknown road.

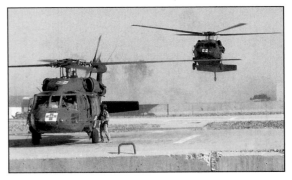

A pair of medevacs land on our concrete helipad.

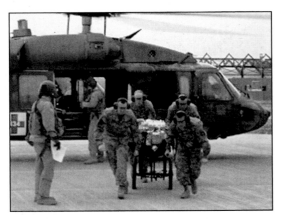

Medics race a wounded soldier into the ER, a trip that took less than a minute.

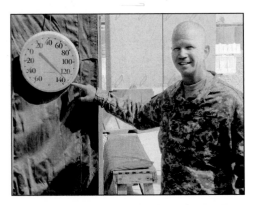

Summer temperatures often hit the mid 130s. We had the luxury of air conditioning. The soldiers in the field did not.

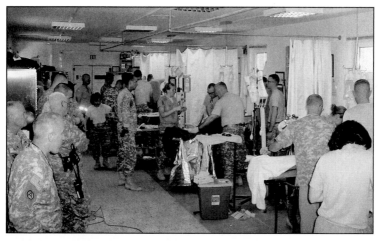

After a series of roadside bombs, our trauma bays filled with the wounded.

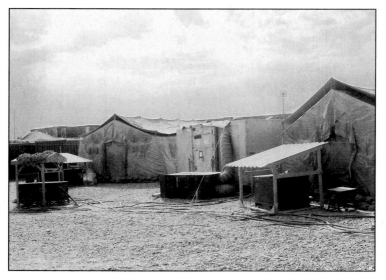

The hospital wasn't much to look at, but the care we provided was top-notch.

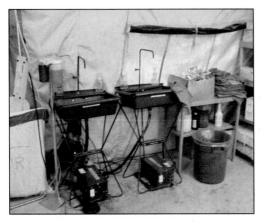

The primitive plastic scrub sinks of the OR.

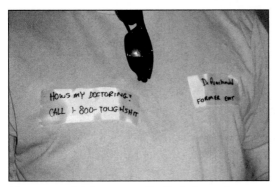

I carried my blood-stained and sweat-soaked cheat sheets everywhere, but never had to use them.

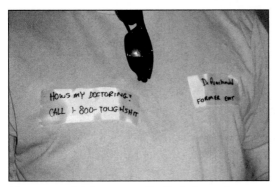

My nametags didn't go over well with the bosses, but our patients loved them.

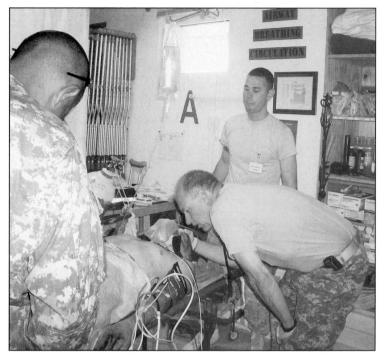

Alpha bay, where the best bedside manner was a calm and reassuring voice.

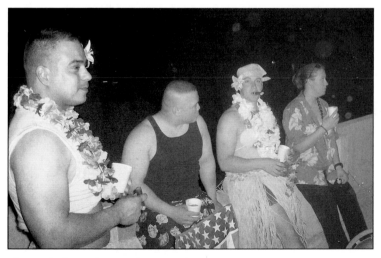

The standard attire for our infamous rooftop parties.

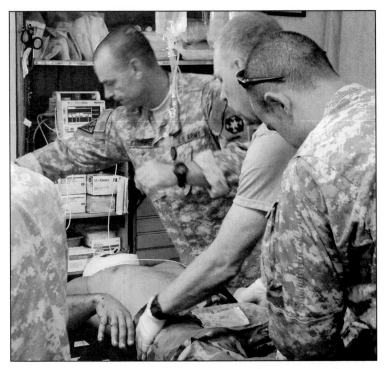

I check the pelvis of a wounded Iraqi soldier while Sergeant Courage works in the background.

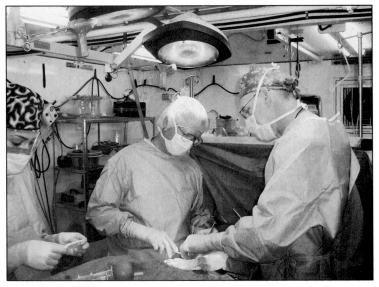

Rick and I perform late-night surgery.

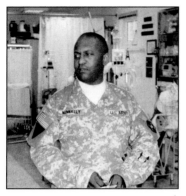

Ian Nunnally, stellar surgeon and forgiving roommate.

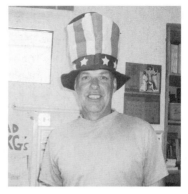

"Uncle Dave" on July 4th, an hour before we were swamped with wounded soldiers.

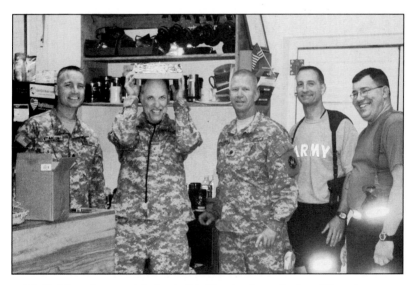

My birthday cake, seconds before it slid off my head onto the floor. We ate it anyway. *(l-r: Bill Stanton, me, Rick Reutlinger, Mike Barron, Gerry Maloney)*

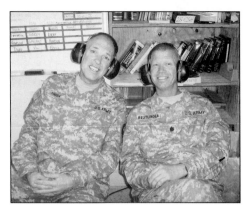

Wearing Mickey Mouse ear protectors, Rick and I
croon off-key our favorite songs for the staff.

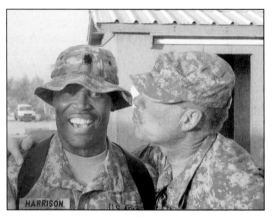

Bernard's farewell kiss. It made a lot of women jealous.

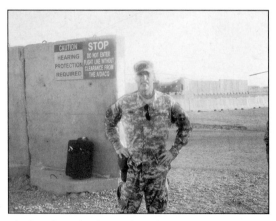

The best day is the day you leave for home.

12

SICK CALL SUNDAY

IKE ANY HOSPITAL, the pace at Paradise could vary from crazy busy to sluggish slow. On the busy ones, we didn't have time to pee, while on slow shifts the medics fought boredom by staging scorpion-versus-camel-spider fights, or by watching slasher movies that drew belly laughs for the fake blood splashing across the screen. A few of the females, and even a couple of males, had taken up knitting and crochet. Instead of war souvenirs, they'd bring home scarves and blankets. You also needed to look both ways before crossing the ER to avoid being run over by the NASCAR-like wheelchair races.

By mid-July, business was on the upswing, with a steady flow of patients and even a few periods where our operating rooms had been open around the clock. I had been designated the official "shit magnet" for the weeks before, the term for the doctor who had the highest number of trauma cases when on duty. It was better than being designated "007"—as in licensed to kill. Make a mistake and you were called Dr. Bond until someone else fouled up and stole the title. Fortunately, our mistakes seemed few and minor—and no patients had suffered from our work. Nonetheless, I didn't want to be introduced as: Bond, Dave Bond.

Our wards get full, then empty as patients are flown to Germany or, if Iraqi, discharged into the local medical system—a health care nightmare we call the kennels. The wards quickly refill and the cycle repeats itself.

Though the majority of patients we'd get were the wounded, I was surprised at the number of everyday medical problems similar to what we saw day to day in the States. Overall, 77 percent of soldiers evacuated to Germany or the United States had noncombat problems that bought them a one-way ticket out of the war. Bad backs, high blood pressure, and bum knees beat shrapnel as the chief reasons combat commanders had trouble keeping their units filled with warm bodies. As a full-service hospital with an oversized welcome mat, we also took care of a lot of contractors. They also had bosses who growled when we had to pull their workers off the schedule because of an ache, pain, or something more serious.

There had been a regular flow of patients with appendicitis, several each week, as well as a steady stream of kidney stones. Both problems were probably due to the searing heat and the fact it was nearly impossible to swill the ten to fifteen big bottles of water needed to head off dehydration, especially for the soldiers who went outside the wire in full battle gear. Migraines were another big-ticket item as well as, of all things, heart attacks. It was the rare soldier who had a heart problem, usually it was overweight contractors in their forties and fifties who smoked like chimneys and ate like pigs at the trough.

Then again, a number of the soldiers we saw would also easily qualify for the cover of *Weight Watchers*. The food here sucked, but there was plenty of it, especially cakes and pies, so that average ten-and-a-half-pound weight gain made the weight control program one of the busiest in the war zone.

Sundays were the worst days in the ER. The sick call clinic was

closed, so in addition to the combat trauma that landed on our helipad, we got the pain-in-the-ass stuff. And this day, Sunday, I drew the
short scalpel, and got to juggle IEDs with constipation. And listen to a
bunch of contractors who suffered from "Acute Ambien Deficiency"
plead for piles of the precious sleeping pills.

It was a far cry from a day filled with the adrenaline-pumping
pressure of trauma cases—not that we wanted trauma cases but the
routine had become torture. So we broke up the monotony of the
Sunday routine by making the diagnosis with the fortune-telling
Magic 8-Ball. When a soldier asked when they'd feel better, we broke
out the ball, gave it a shake, and hoped it didn't return an answer of
"Outlook not so good." In that case, we were forced to shake, and
shake, and shake again until we got an answer that eased anxiety. And
for the stubborn "Ask again later," all we could say was: go to sick call
tomorrow if you want a look into your future.

Another tactic was to use libido in place of drugs to affect a cure.
Think of it as alternative medicine in a war zone. Nonmedicinally
natural. For a male with a nonserious case of "something that won't
kill you," we pulled out the latest edition of the New England Patriots
cheerleader calendar for a curative leaf-through; the females got the
NYC Firemen of the Year, bare-chested edition. Or we simply pulled
out a picture of Bernard.

But this day, before commuting the quarter mile to work, I had
my weekly business meeting during breakfast with Rick. Basically, it
was a time for two grumpy old men to clear the air and start the week
on a fresh footing.

Rick had the first item on the agenda.

"You know, I think you curse too much. So the least you can do is
give my virginal ears some peace on the Lord's day."

I rolled my eyes.

"What the hell are you talking about? You curse, too."

"But not on Sundays."

"Bullshit."

"How about 'male cattle manure' instead? It would make God happy."

I almost spit out my coffee.

"I'm sure God is really worried about my language. And I'm really sure God wants me to say stupid stuff like 'male cattle manure.'"

Rick gave me a serious look. "I bet you can't do it. In fact, I will give you twenty bucks if you can get through your shift without cursing. However, if you fail, you owe me a dollar a curse. Plus, you can forget about lunch."

"You're on. Today. Only."

"Thanks, Dave."

"You bet . . . penis cranium."

He did the verbal translation and gave me a nasty scowl.

"Okay, Dave, your turn to moan. How did I bother you this week?"

"You're ugly."

With that final insult, I grabbed my tray and raced out the chow hall to face my day of hell, or in this case, let's call it "heck."

I walked in just as the medics were throwing out the first patient of the day. It was a soldier who said his back had been sore for a month. The medic absentmindedly rolled a pencil off the desk. Sergeant Sore Back easily bent over to pick it up. A nice gesture that determined his prescription: You can wait. Go to sick call tomorrow.

The next guy wanted to quit smoking. A surefire ticket to better health in a war zone. The chief medic asks for his cigarettes, which are then thrown on the floor and stomped on. "Don't buy any more before sick call tomorrow."

Our third winner said he had a painful nostril.

"I have a sore inside my nose that's been there for three weeks and I can't get it to go away."

"How did the sore get there?"

"I was picking my nose. And every time I pick my nose it gets sorer."

"Well, here's the latest clinical research on a cure: stop picking your nose. Now get out."

Sounds brutal but there was a good reason to keep the not-very-urgent cases from causing a traffic jam in our ER: we needed to keep our stretchers open for the more serious cases that showed up with little warning. Within minutes, the radioman stuck his head in and confirmed that "Please come back tomorrow" was indeed a wise policy.

"Business coming. One urgent on a litter. Burns from blast. Estimate fifteen mikes."

Mikes-minutes-months-millenniums. I lived in a world of milspeak and secret codes. I chuckled. *This must be Gerry's idea of heaven.* Then I quickly felt bad when I realized there was a wounded human on the other end of that chuckle.

Twelve mikes later, the medics rolled in our patient. From a distance, he didn't look so hot. He had a tube in his throat and the medics were bent at 90-degree angles over the stretcher as it squeaked rapidly across the cracked linoleum.

We did some quick calculations: burns over 60 percent of his body. Not good. Singed mustache and soot around the mouth— inhalation injuries to the lungs. He'd also suffered blast injuries: some of his bones were pointing north, others south. I gently pulled on his arm to open a path to wiggle my stethoscope onto his chest. The skin from elbow to wrist pulled off in one long solid piece—like a glove being removed. I was afraid to tug on anything else for fear it would just slide off into my hands.

I took my time with a portable ultrasound, his belly was becoming increasingly firm and tight, and the scan confirmed blood leaking inside the abdominal cavity as the reason why.

The complexity of his wounds swallowed a chunk of time. From exam to X-rays to treatment, it took close to a half an hour before I was ready to turn the patient over to Ian. I was glad he'd drawn the surgical on-call straw for the day. He'd need to find, then fix, the source of the bleeding in his abdomen—I suspected a chunk of shrapnel plowed its way into something important. But Ian was also the best guy we had in burn care, so he'd start removing the worst of the crisp tissue, then repeat the process over the next few days.

Then Bill would have his turn, setting and straightening crooked bones. Finally, our internist would fiddle with the respirator to find the right settings that would push needed air into the scorched lungs. That, and finding the right antibiotics to protect a now fragile body from infection.

I actually thought the guy would make it . . . if he were an American. But he was an Iraqi soldier, so even if we saved him today, he'd be transferred to an Iraqi hospital where the care was so bad the odds pointed to a quick death.

As he was wheeled to surgery, the doors to the ER were roped open to let in fresh air. Blood has a sticky sweet smell—often more nauseating to see than smell—but the odor of a bad burn is something else. It attacks the nose and throat and won't let go. It attaches itself to your nostrils, and at times, like today, leaves a horrible taste in your mouth. No amount of brushing or gargling can cleanse away the bitter tang of charred human flesh.

Now that our Iraqi soldier was gone, we screeched from bedlam to boredom. The next few hours morphed into a blenderized mix of the routine: ingrown toenails, infected bug bites, a slip and fall in the shower that resulted in a nasty gash to the back of the head—a wound easily and quickly stapled together, to the surprise of the soldier who owned the head.

"You're going to do what to my head?"

"Staple it," I answered.

"What do you mean staple it?"

"What I said. Staples. Little metal things that attach piles of papers. Make believe the cut on your head is a loose pile of papers. We're going to staple the papers back together."

"No you're not."

Snap. Snap. Snap. Snap.

"Just did. If you need any further assistance with cuts, wounds, stationery, or office supplies, please remember we're here. And by all means, tell your friends. Thanks for shopping with us."

I looked up in time to see Rick standing over by the nurse's desk. There were murmurs and whispers floating in the area.

"No, sir, he hasn't said one dirty word all day."

"Y'all sure? He's got a potty mouth."

"Clean, sir. He's got the tongue of an angel today."

I strolled over toward the buzzing and glared at Rick.

"We've got a special on staples today. Need any? Like on your lips?"

"How's your day, Dave?" he said with an innocent look.

"Just swell. I'm swell. Having a peachy day. Dad-gum it, things just couldn't get better."

"Okay, buddy, here's your lunch for the day. Just remember, I've got spies everywhere."

I was famished. The second he left, I popped open the Styrofoam container and unwrapped my noontime fare. Chili with onions. Turkey on white with onions. Chips with artificial onion dip. A piece of cake with sliced onions on top. I hate onions. Despise onions. In my world, a weapon of mass destruction was an onion bomb.

"You mother—" I skidded to a stop, looked up, and saw eager eyes peering my way.

"—of blessed Jesus our Lord. What a saint. He brought me an appetizer, main course, and dessert. What a pal."

Disappointment rose across the room. Thought they had me. What was this, a conspiracy? I thought the medics were on my side! I bet Reutlinger had promised them a slice of the winning bet if I slipped and blasphemed.

My thoughts of killing Rick were interrupted by the bang and whoosh of the opening door. It was another radio message.

"Badblood is giving us a heads-up on a big one. Sounds like up to fifteen wounded coming in."

All heads jerked up. "How many?" gets asked by several of us simultaneously. One-fiver is the repeated answer.

I swung my boots off my makeshift desk and looked over at Major Boutin, the head nurse of the day.

"Roger, that's a ton. We need every live body to get over here. Or at least give everybody a heads-up."

"I don't think we need to call a mascal until we get more info— sounds like it's a question mark if we're even getting anybody." Mascal stood for mass casualties, a situation that required all hands report to the hospital.

"I know, but you know what fifteen wounded would do to this place if they all fall out of the sky at once."

"Agree. But let's wait a couple," he answered.

So we sat and squirmed. The Styrofoam containers with our lunches got tossed into big plastic trashcans and some of the medics started to make up the trauma bays—putting out IVs and trauma packs. Nervous stomachs and anxious bladders sent a few off to the latrine. The slow tick of the wall clock could be heard above the low growl of small talk in the room.

The door swung back open.

"Number now at fourteen. Destination unknown. Could be us, Balad, or Baghdad, or none of the above. There's a lot of chatter on the line. But they're starting to move some people out."

I walked over to Roger.

"I think maybe the compromise is a heads-up. No one needs to come over but it might be a good idea to just let people know there's a possibility. Maybe hold off a nap or a workout for the next half hour."

Roger slowly nodded. "Okay. I'll put out pages to everyone. Tell them NOT to come, but there is a small chance we could be real busy soon. But let's play it safe and let them know we'll page them again when we hear more."

The surgeons, backup docs, respiratory therapists, nursing staff,

X-ray, lab, adminsitrators all got paged to be available. The text on the pager was clear: *Potential mascal. Do not come. Repeat, do not come. Expect zero to fourteen patients. Further info to follow.*

The clock continued to tick slower than our hearts. I realized I was in a T-shirt with a joke nametag. The tape that said "Dr. Frankenstein" got crumpled and tossed in the trash.

Ten long minutes passed when the doors finally banged open again.

"Stand down. No casualties coming our way."

Roger quickly sent out a page telling everyone to relax. But within minutes, a three-man parade of stooges began.

One by one, the administrators marched in. Each red-faced and spewing venom. Their separate speeches had the subtlety and tact of a hand grenade.

"What the hell are you people doing! You can't scare the hell out of everyone for something that's not going to happen."

Followed by: "Are you people stupid or something? You don't call a mascal when no one comes. You're wasting my time."

Followed by: "I can't believe what just happened. You page every goddamn person in this place for something that's not happening. We came running over from lunch because of these pages. You better get some counseling on why and when to page personnel."

A few poison stares came my way, but most of the hatred was pointed at Roger. He sputtered out a few words of reason, but I think he was caught off guard by the viciousness of the attacks. The diatribes only lasted a few minutes, but each violated a cardinal rule of command: never embarrass an officer in front of his troops. And Roger went down hard in front of a large group of medics and nurses. I sat by quietly—too quietly—as the scenes played out. I should have stuck up for Roger—after all, I was the one afraid of a deluge of wounded, but failed him by staying silent.

As the last screamer left, I meandered over to Roger and asked if he'd step outside for a second.

The wind was starting to whip up, the tongue of fire sandblasting our faces as I apologized.

"I should have spoken up. It was me who asked you to page everyone. I just don't understand why they went nuts—it was only a heads-up."

The Zen-like officer gave me a serene look.

"We did the right thing. You know, Jack Twomey would have done it, too. One thing he taught me was to drill and be ready. And never take chances with the troops. If it was his son coming in, he'd say we did right."

"What do you mean?"

"Jack's son is a marine. And he's here in country right now. Heaven help us if his kid ever came in, but we'd be ready because Jack has been saying since we got here that we *had better* be ready in case *his* kid ever does come through the door. That's why we were ready today. If it wasn't his kid, it was someone else's kid. So screw those guys—they don't know anything about patients."

Now things made sense. Jack Twomey was a quiet man—often quiet to a point where at times I felt uncomfortable. But if I were in his boots, I'd be quiet and serious, too. Unlike those who sat and worried at home thousands of miles away from their child in the war, Jack was right next door, and it would be horrible to be notified that your son had been wounded by personally seeing his face lolling on a stretcher. Christ, he must swallow his heart every time the radio squawks.

Roger's words and demeanor lowered my temperature a few degrees and the steam from my ears slowly dissipated into the desert heat. But I was still pissed at the Three Stooges who had yelled at us, and wondered if there was a path down the road to payback for Moe, Larry, and Curly. I didn't need to worry about getting my hands dirty, though. As I walked back into the ER, one of the medics pulled me aside and said, "Don't you worry, sir. Those guys have been dicks all year, and a bunch of us figure it's time to have a little fun. You watch, sir."

I sighed and shook my head—sometimes you wondered which

side of the war some of the administrators were on. I'd step back and let medic-karma take its course.

At the stroke of seven, Mike marched in to take over the reins. I grabbed my weapon from the lockbox and headed to dinner. The bulk of the group was already there but mostly quiet, with little of the usual mealtime banter. Last week was a bugger; this week hadn't started any easier. Everyone looked tired. Our mood was further soured by the news that some of our friends, active duty doctors from the 82nd Airborne, had just been told to unpack their bags. Originally slated to head home in a few weeks, the group's homecoming was now delayed to October. Another twelve-month deployment extended to fifteen. The stress on the troops was reaching epic proportions.

We took a nighttime walk back to the hospital to check e-mail and give a quick call home. All quiet on that front. As we felt our darkened way across the gravel back to barracks, Rick said, "You know, I didn't think you could do it. Looks like I owe you twenty bucks."

"Keep it," I said. "There's nothing to spend it on, anyway." I think I had gone through a whole $4.32 at the PX since we arrived, mainly on shaving cream and deodorant. "You can buy me a beer when we get home."

Two tired men made their way up the stairs that night. I'd flip a movie into my computer and Rick would read another book. At least until I snuck down a flight of stairs at five minutes to twelve. I banged on Rick's plywood door like the barracks were on fire, and then hid around the corner. When he barged out of his room in bare feet, he never saw the slippery tray of onion-filled foods I had retrieved from the trashcan in the ER. He slipped and slid like a man doing a drunken jig.

"Shit. Bastard. Damn. I'm going to kill you, asshole."

I just calmly turned and walked down the dimly lit hallway.

"Hey, Oklahoma boy. Watch your mouth, it's still Sunday. But I gotta admit, I do love the way you dance, honey."

As his scowl melted into a grin, I tossed him a final good night.

"Sleep well, onion-head."

13

DANTE'S INFIRMARY

(They picked him up in the grass where he had lain two days in the
rain with a piece of shrapnel in his lungs.)
COME to me only with playthings now . . .
A picture of a singing woman with blue eyes
Standing at a fence of hollyhocks, poppies and sunflowers . . .
Or an old man I remember sitting with children telling stories
Of days that never happened anywhere in the world . . .

A FRIEND FROM MY Reserve unit back home e-mailed me a poem from Carl Sandburg the week before. It was written during World War I and described a soldier who was wounded, taken to a field hospital . . . then dreamed of only beautiful and peaceful things as he awaited surgery and transport home. It's called "Murmurings in a Field Hospital."

The poem made me think of how frightened the wounded were when they came in—you could always see it in their eyes—as well as how frightened we were to take care of the wounded. I wondered if they could see it in our eyes. I wondered if they heard the murmurings in a combat hospital, like we did.

As I read the e-mail, I was scraping small bits of flesh off my pants legs near my ankles and getting ready to pour a bottle of peroxide on my boots to dissolve away the bloodstains. Even when clean, I wondered how much gore, and memories of gore, I would bring home with me.

I was finally at a point where I wasn't too worried about my skills, whether it was caring for a guy whose limbs had been shredded or whose eardrums were ruptured and bleeding thanks to an IED. But when done . . . Jesus. You were forced to watch a mental rerun of your every move and decision, and your movie snack wasn't popcorn, instead an overflowing tub of adrenaline-soaked fear.

The night before, I thought a lot about breathing, not a subject I would even consider worthy of a fleeting thought back home. A gunshot wound made me think about all the ways we talked about "a breath." You take one, you lose one, steal one, hold one, waste one, save one, run out of . . . the combinations went on and on. And those combinations dominated a corner of my mind as I watched a young soldier heave for air after being shot. As I did my exam, I couldn't shake the thought of what his lungs were trying to do. A simple act that we don't think very much about. Yet for this kid, I prayed he'd take another. And another. And another. And he did.

Funny, I don't think my heart started galloping, at least to where I noticed it, until I sat down after the case had been handed off to one of the surgeons. Did I do well? Did I screw anything up? In most circumstances, I would never know. In fact, a good outcome was when we saved a soldier and shipped him out within twenty-four hours— never to hear about him again. I was just one blurred face in a bustling mix of people who would care for him over the next months or years. I had simply been one of the first, and probably one of the forgotten. But I could live with that—as long as he lived long enough to have a chance to forget me.

The wounds of this war were certainly vicious, but no worse than the ones my father witnessed, or the ones suffered by the soldier who lay in a field for two days during World War I, or for that matter, any war since someone decided to invent war.

I knew people back home saw and heard about the deaths and the wounds, but on a screen or in writing it was all sanitized and sterile. Just numbers. Statistics often selfishly used, by some, for political arguments about the rights or wrongs of this war. They didn't see, feel, or smell what a broken body is like up close and personal. And they didn't have to make the decisions we did. Save the arm? Save the leg? Save the soldier?

We had only seconds to decide what would define the rest of someone's life, and in turn, the lives of the loved ones who would care for them. With all of the advances in military medicine, we played by a new set of rules, and with them came a new set of dilemmas. We saw soldiers who would have quickly died on the battlefield in wars past; in Iraq they came to us maimed, blinded, or with traumatic brain injuries. Save them with their horrific injuries or let them die peacefully? For us, the dilemma was no dilemma: the unspoken rule was save them every time. And we would work ourselves to the grave if it meant getting them home to family.

As for the war itself, we didn't have arguments or discussions. There was no desire, or for that matter, energy. We were too busy trying not to slip and fall in the bloody puddles on the floor. And when our workdays were done, we sat together like a family at dinner and talked about beautiful and peaceful things. Two months into our time here at Dante's Infirmary, and there hadn't been one single hot word between us. We often would speak of family, baseball, a frosty cold beer spilling over the lip of a tall glass. *Bring us playthings.* We were wounded by what we did and what we saw.

But no more than those we cared for. A few days before, I was talking to a grimy sergeant who accompanied a wounded soldier from a firefight in Baquba. I looked at his arms and legs and realized he had tourniquets loosely in place around all four limbs. So did the rest of his squad.

"Doc, we know we're going to get hit one of these days. Better to have the tourniquets on ahead of time. All we've got to do is tighten them up if something bad happens."

He chuckles grimly. "Might save you some work, sir."

This kid was a war machine who lived by the *Be Prepared* credo of a Boy Scout.

All I could do was shake my head at him, and at the others. Many others.

There was a group we'd come to know well on the night shift. We called them our "frequent fliers." It seemed like they came in at least once a week after being blown up. They were a convoy security team who weaved in and out of slow-moving trains of supply trucks. The team had high-tech equipment to detect roadside bombs—maybe that's what kept them from hitting the big ones—but it seemed like they had hit more than their share of little ones lately. One guy had been in six times within the last month, three times within the last ten days. Not a scratch, just nagging headaches.

"Buddy, you are an IED magnet. Ever thought about taking a little break?"

"No can do, Doc. Not enough people. Can't stay home while the rest are riding the roads."

"One more visit and you've got enough points for an upgrade to first class and a nicer stretcher."

We gently touched each other on our sleeves and said no more.

I wondered how long he could keep winning the IED lotto before his luck ran out.

The rest of that particular night was a welcome quiet. I grabbed the stretcher in Delta bay, swung my feet up, and conked until the sun rose and the coffee perked. No foo-foo that day—it was pure high-test, God bless the night crew.

I grabbed an old sandwich from the fridge and walked over to morning rounds, pissed that the sandman in Iraq was truly the sandman. My eyes had quickly filled up with a bunch of gritty granules during the short walk.

Our group stood circled as we went through the motions of discussing a few patients, then perked up when it came time for some official business.

Colonel Quick was succinct as he faced the group.

"I want to make sure everyone has their body armor and masks close at hand at the hospital. If you've got them in your room, bring them back and keep them in the ER or OR. They shouldn't be there in the first place. No exceptions. There have been some chlorine attacks in the area and I want us to be prepared."

We hadn't been hit with choking chlorine gas yet, but the word on the street was a suicide bomber was going to ram a chlorine-filled truck bomb through the southeast gate, the one closest to the hospital and virtually just outside our door. The explosion of a bomb would be bad enough; the suffocating release of the gas would kill many more.

The next warning was more chilling: the bad guys really wanted to get their hands on a female nurse—grab her—then make a throat-cutting video. There were a few nervous chuckles when we were told we males weren't high on the wish list.

"Let's not forget this is a real war," added Quick.

After rounds, Rick and I meandered back toward the barracks, playing our version of Kick the Can, except here we use a large rock.

"You have a lot of rumors when you were in Afghanistan?" I asked as we kicked our way across the compound.

"Tons. Mainly that we ate children. You know, a lot of kids stepped on mines left over from the Russians, but the parents didn't want to bring them in to us. At least until they had bad infections or something. It was always too late, man."

"Crazy stuff here, too. You ever hear the one about our sunglasses? They give us X-ray vision so we can see through women's clothes. Our bullets are radioactive and what the candy guys toss out to kids is poison."

The last one brought back a memory of a trip to an Iraqi school in 2004 and giving handfuls of candy to a swirling mob of grade-schoolers. They looked and acted just like American kids grabbing and kicking and fighting each other for the sweets—until their teachers scurried out.

"*Tawaqqafa! Tawaqqafa!*" Stop! Stop!

They took the candy away, told us it would be eaten later—but we knew otherwise. They were just little kids caught in the middle of a war. As we looked at the teachers in the bright sunlight, our eyes protected by tinted goggles, they turned away quickly. The men in the group thanked us and shooed us away.

"Going to lunch soon?" Rick asked.

I snapped back to the present.

"Only if you drive me in the surrey with the fringe on top."

"The heat burned off all of the fringe. It's a bald surrey."

"Then forget it, I wouldn't be caught dead in that thing. I'll catch you for dinner; remember I've got nights again."

As we entered the barracks, we looked at each other and rubbed our eyes. Did we just see what we think we saw? A ghostlike apparition of a nurse in a Victoria's Secret nighty, tiptoeing down our hallway.

"Isn't it a little early for afternoon delight?" Rick asked.

"I guess it's never too early if you've got the time and the privacy."

"Hell, the high point of my day is taking a good dump. I think my grapefruits do a nice job loosening the old plumbing."

I just looked at Rick as we walked in the door. Sex versus poop. Which becomes more important as we age? I was afraid of the answer.

I trudged up the stairs and into the Love Shack, said hi to our pinups, then promptly passed out from exhaustion.

I slept the day away and when 6:30 finally rolled around, I was in the middle of a dream where I was trapped in an earthquake, and it was flinging my body like a rag doll. I was scared shitless and when I opened my eyes, they quickly focused on a hideous monster face. It was Rick, standing over my body, shaking me awake. Startled, I bit off a scream.

"Christ, is this the face your wife wakes up to every morning? She must take antinausea medicine before bed."

"Hey, douche. You've got to be at the hospital in a half hour. Get your ass moving."

I was just about to yell at him for letting me oversleep when I saw a couple of containers of food on my chair.

"I figured you needed your beauty sleep," he said, "but then I realized you needed to wake up before next January. Your ugliness ain't going to be cured this deployment."

The folding chair was overflowing with a banquet of a stewlike mixture of stringy meat on noodles, a corn dog, and a couple of sandwiches. Plus three cans of Harika Tat.

I mumbled a thanks, then grabbed my crumpled uniform off the floor.

"Anything up?" I asked as I shook every thread of clothing like a disco dancer on speed.

"Not much. Lots of crap in the air so we were on red most of the day. The Tongue of Fire was extra hot so I couldn't work out. Would have shriveled up like a dead worm on a Mississippi sidewalk. I'll stop by later."

Rick said a quick goodbye to Edith, Ethel, and Isabel as he walked out the door. He never patted or rubbed their butts like some of our visitors did. He was a good husband in love and war.

The ER was set on medium-high when I walked in. Mike had his hands full with a hodgepodge of cases; a couple of guys who were shaken in an IED blast, a young soldier with a migraine, and the mystery case of a contractor who couldn't move the left side of his face. The diagnosis was either a stroke or Bell's palsy. When I told Mike to shove off, he just shook his head.

"Nah, I'm okay. Just got a little bit more to do. A couple of notes to put in the computer."

Even though he had every right to walk out the door at change of shift, he always stayed. Mike knew how hard it was to take over a patient in midstream and never screwed me. For that matter, neither did Gerry. It was an informal rule among us.

Mike didn't get out until well after eight, missing dinner. "Oh, I've got some energy bars to eat." In the meantime, I just sat around with my feet up, waiting for the next new patient.

And I waited. And waited. I hated nights like this. Sometimes I would go outside and sweep the sidewalk—a great surprise for Sergeant Courage in the morning—or go lift rusty weights and barbells at our makeshift exercise patio next to the OR tent.

You could never relax, always worrying something bad was going to attack as soon as you put your guard down. Get lulled into a pinch of relaxation, that was the time you might screw up or make a bad decision.

That night, just minutes after the clock struck midnight, I faced a decision that could have gone bad.

He was an insurgent, flown in by chopper and rushed to Alpha bay by the medics. Had to be in his mid to late twenties, a hard stubble of beard on his face. A blood mustache. Clothes dirty and ragged, cut off quickly as the gurney was wheeled from the helipad to the ER, now piled in a heap on the floor.

He seemed to be snoring, a bad sign, which usually signifies the struggled breathing of brain damage. The right side of his skull was expanding outward, giving him a cartoonish appearance. The flight medic told me the insurgent had been shot while planting IEDs. Without a scratch anywhere on his body, and an oddly shaped skull, the sharpshooter's aim must have been true—a perfect shot to the back of the head.

I expected a mess so I double-gloved. Gently lifting his head, I slid my hand underneath. My fingers were quickly lost in a crater of mush. As I pulled them out, a slimy mass of gray brain tissue stuck to my gloves. One of the medics got nauseated and left the room—I couldn't blame her.

I couldn't find an exit wound, which meant the bullet still had to be somewhere inside the cranium, so I called in X-ray to snap a quick picture—the shadowy film showed the sharp outline of a bullet sitting smack in the middle of the brain. No way this guy was going to make it. Yet he still had a heartbeat, and as irregular as they were, breaths continued to force their way into struggling lungs. Official protocol said we had to pull out the stops and save him, or at least keep him alive until we could fly him down to the neurosurgeons in Balad.

Following Abu Ghraib, the rules regarding the care of insurgents were increasingly strict. We were ordered to give the best of care, then our work was microreviewed after the fact to make sure. There was even a rumor that insurgents who died in our care were flown to the U.S. for an autopsy. We knew they made it as far as Baghdad, but Dover, Delaware?

Out came the drugs, IVs with life-sustaining blood, and the imaginary book of medical miracles. The drugs were injected as fast as thumbs could squeeze the syringes, the blood poured back out as fast as it poured in, and the book of miracles had nothing but empty pages.

"Let's call up the birds," I said. "This guy needs to make a quick trip to Balad."

We'd kept him alive just to let him die somewhere else. It was clear the bullet didn't just plow straight into the brain—it had to hit the inside walls of the skull and ricochet like a lethal Ping-Pong ball from corner to corner, destroying brain tissue with every bounce. He was going to die—the question was when and where.

One of the medics tapped my sleeve.

"Sir, we've got to give the helicopters about a fifteen-minute heads-up. Is this an urgent?"

The answer was obviously yes, the guy had been shot in the head.

"No."

"They also say the weather is a little iffy, but they can fly in it. They'll need two birds for this run. Plus a flight nurse for the patient."

"Whose turn?" I asked.

A voice came from behind.

"That would be me, sir." Lieutenant Ward stood looking at me. The whole team stood looking at me.

"Well, saddle up and let's prep this guy for the flight."

No hesitation.

"Yes, sir." Yes, sirs followed all around.

Portable oxygen, monitors, and emergency drugs were bundled for the flight.

"Let's wrap that head up nice and tight with some clean dressings. When you're ready, get the flight line on the phone, and move this guy down the road."

There was a bustle of activity. I looked at the monitors still attached to our guy. Blood pressure lower. Heart racing at 160, but still regular. Respirations labored and irregular but he was breathing on his own. He was fighting death. Hard. But he was starting to lose ground.

Then I looked over at Lieutenant Ward. First name Warren. Great nurse, great guy. From Ohio. Three kids. He'd be rocking-and-rolling in cramped quarters with a dying insurgent, and if the guy died on the flight, it would be Ward's head on the platter. Plus he'd be going up in sand-filled skies with lousy visibility—him *and* the flight crew. And then there was the extra crew of the escort chopper. They'd be thirty seconds behind in the same bad weather. Throw in the possibility of getting shot at, and the risks were enormous.

I stepped away from the stretcher for a minute, and thought hard as I watched each member of the staff scurry to bundle up the insurgent for the flight.

"Hey, everybody. I need your opinion." I looked slowly into each person's eyes. "Does everyone agree we've done everything we could?"

A few seconds of hesitation with a few stolen glances at each other. Then came a flurry of head nods and positive murmurs all around.

"Does anyone think this guy has any chance at all?"

Head shakes and mumbled murmurs to that question.

"Then stand down. Mr. Ward, take off your shit. Call the birds, tell them to go back to bed. This is a no-go."

I stepped outside and had a heated argument with myself. Another classic paradox in Paradise. The odds of something bad happening during the flight were high. And even if the flight made it safely, would Ward be delivering a dead body? But then again, the guy was still alive. And deserved care. Yet, he was going to die, neurosurgery or no neurosurgery. Then, what about the official protocol for the medical care of insurgents? Hell, screw the protocol, it was bullshit. The "cover your ass" rules of the Army weren't worth the life of one of my people, let alone the six Americans that would make the trip. They all had families. They needed to make it home alive.

The argument ended in a draw; there was no right answer.

I went back inside. A couple of staff members scurried to meet me.

"Sir, you know the rules. The protocols. They're strict."

"Here's the deal. I am the one who made this decision. No one else did. Consider this an official order: he stays. So do our people. If anyone comes bitching about the breach in protocol—send them to me. You're all off the hook."

A sense of relief coated everyone in the room. They didn't need to look up the word "futile" in the dictionary, they were seeing it in real life heaving for air on a stretcher.

I owed the medics and nurses—each and every one. These people had given me their all during my rotation here, saving my skin more times than I'd like to admit. And I was going to make sure Warren Ward and friends made it home to their families.

For the next two hours, we stood, sat, leaned, and watched. The insurgent slowly continued to weaken, his body surrendering to the inevitable. His pupils were fixed and dilated, he didn't respond to anything we did. We gave him morphine in case he felt any pain on his journey to death but I don't think it was needed. An EKG finally showed a flat line—no pulse, no respiration. We ran an extra copy to give to the authorities. Then called the morgue.

Many of the medics went outside to smoke cigarettes. And as each burst of sandy wind whipped through the dark sky, Warren Ward slowly looked up and shook his head.

The insurgent took a long time to die, maybe too long. I expected to have my ass handed to me on a plate the next day, but no one said a word. Not that day, or the rest of our days. It was the best medical decision I had made in my time at the CSH. It was also the first time in my Army career I had ever actually given an official order. I was happy about the former, proud of the latter.

Some say all human life is equal. Yet I valued the lives of my people more than that of a man who planted bombs. I hoped my people all made it home safely, and that I was, in some way, part of making that happen.

14

DEATH OF AN AMERICAN SOLDIER

HOW COME IT took so much time to get the damned blood?"

The question came from one of our nurse anesthetists.

"We hurried as fast as we could. I have to account for every unit of blood that leaves the lab and make sure it's what's been ordered by the ER."

The lab director looked hurt as she answered.

"Well, it still should have come faster," came the reply.

"And I want to know what took so long to get the portable X-ray into position."

That accusation arose from a different voice near the rear of the tent.

The defense angrily answered from the front row.

"It was there in plenty enough time. We were just waiting until we were cleared to enter the bay."

The verbal pitchforks had been flying for close to an hour as we stuffed ourselves into a musty tent to dissect the worst case of our deployment: the first American soldier to die on our watch. He was killed the day before, but instead of healing, time was salt in our wound. A day after his death, we all continued to sink deeper into the quicksand of depression.

Now came the question I was hoping we'd never have to answer, especially after busting our humps to save insurgents. How would we react after losing our first American?

Colonel Quick was a silent referee. He sat quietly at the front of the tent, rocking back in his chair, peering over his glasses as a collection of the hospital staff pointed imaginary fingers of blame around the tent. As for the doctors, we just sat there, our fingers silently pointed at ourselves yet offering nary a word aloud. In reality, there was enough blame to go around, none of it deserved. There was nothing anyone could have done to save this kid.

Ironically, the day of his death had started on a high note, with us feeling pretty good about ourselves. We were in a groove—a nice rhythm where we were working well together. We knew our jobs. Knew our limitations. And who we could count on to bail us out when we were in a medical fix. We joked at breakfast over the perks of life in the Army: free food, free drop-off laundry service, and no traffic jams; hell, we walked to work every morning. Even better was the absence of insurance companies. We lived in a world of minimal paperwork where if we wanted a test or treatment, there was no second-guessing or pleading over a telephone.

We were even getting the hang of attacking the monotony of the menu. While Rick still ate his pile of daily grapefruits, I wanted to patent my breakfast invention: "Corn Krispie Cap'n Cocoa Loops"— an overflowing concoction that, when drowned in a carton of warm Turkish milk, tasted like a bowl of dirty socks. But at least it had taste, a surefire selling point in a place like Iraq.

The rest of the breakfast discussions centered on the upcoming cases of the morning: the cleaning out of wounds in the operating room—basically a power wash of day-old gunshot and shrapnel holes; weaning some guys off ventilators to see if they could breathe on their own; and finally, trying to kick an especially nasty insurgent out of the ICU and transfer his ass to a prison hospital in Baghdad. This guy was a real prick. He'd had several hours of life-saving surgery done by Ian and Bill but when he woke up, his thanks were delivered with a thick load of spittle in the face of the nurse trying to change his dressings. So now he wore a "spit mask"—a surgical mask taped tightly so the only place the spit could travel would be back onto his own face.

As we finished breakfast, a tug on the sleeve brought some good news: Bill said he had hustled up a couple of baseball mitts and a softball. We'd head over to an open field after lunch and play a little All-American catch.

In the meantime, we all had work to do. I wasn't on the schedule, but figured I would spend my morning helping wherever help was needed. My first stop was an overflowing ER. Every bay was filled, every curtain drawn. Mike was running his ass off, evaluating patients and flinging orders in every direction.

I threw out a generic "Which bay do you need me in?" to the room.

The answer from the middle of chaos was a classic.

"Hey, who's in Alpha, what's in Bravo, and I don't know who's in Charlie. But I don't give a damn."

I was now working with Drs. Abbott and Costello.

The only thing in the coffeepot was the overcooked, burnt residue of the morning's brew—no one had time to make a fresh pot and a thick skin of dead coffee lined the bottom of the carafe. I poured in some water, swirled it around, and drank the foul concoction as quickly as my throat could swallow it, just in time for an Iraqi policeman to be stretchered in.

The Iraqi cops were an odd lot. By day, many played cop for the fledgling government; by night, they changed into their insurgent clothes and planted roadside bombs. They often wore a patchwork of shirts and pants; sometimes the only official piece of uniform was an armband that said "Police" in Arabic lettering. No matter, we were an equal opportunity hospital: show up at the door and you got care.

Usually the wounded came by chopper; after being shot in the chest, this guy was simply thrown into the back of a Humvee and quickly trucked over bumpy roads to the CSH. It was the kind of wound that distinguished the Iraqis from Americans; they didn't have body armor and a sniper shot was usually aimed at the chest. Americans, on the other hand, were targeted differently, with unprotected necks, armpits, and groins the targets of choice.

We hustled a soldier with a minor IED headache out of Delta bay as I took the combat medic's report. The displaced soldier looked flustered until he saw the stretcher with a bloody shirt and the chest inside it heaving for air. He scooted quickly to a folding chair at the end of the room, knowing it would be a while until his turn came.

The report was succinct with little emotion.

"Gunshot wound to right thorax. Sucking chest wound. Chest tube with flutter in place. Vital signs up and down. Some other dings and dents but nothing too serious except the chest."

The medics and nurses went to work. After more than a year of trauma care, they had seen it all, and needed little direction. Their requests for IVs, blood, pain medication, and antibiotics often sounded more like "this is what we're doing and we're only asking because the rules say we need to." Fine with me—it made things move more quickly and allowed me to concentrate on the big picture. I usually answered them with quick nods of the head or monosyllabic "Yeps."

I checked the Iraqi from head to toe. The only thing I could find was a bright red eye staring at me from the right side of his chest; it was the hole where the bullet entered. When we rolled the patient onto his side, I did a quick exam—no open holes in the back, so the bullet was still somewhere deep inside. The tube in his chest acted like an oversized straw, sucking a steady flow of bright red blood out of the area around the now collapsed lung. I paged Rick and Bernard—this guy needed to go to the OR before he bled to death. I would scrub in to help.

With a deft swipe of the scalpel, Bernard opened the chest while Rick spread the ribs to isolate the bleed. On the surface of the skin, the wound didn't look like much—but when the bullet entered the chest, it hit a rib. The bump sent the bullet tumbling, tearing and mangling tissue as it traveled deep into the lung.

"I think the lower lobe is done for, guys," Bernard said as he surveyed the inside of the bloody chest cavity.

Rick peered into the mass of bloody tissue.

"It's hamburger, Bernard. I don't think you can isolate the bleeders."

"What do you think, Dave?"

"Wedge resection?" I answered.

"Correct-a-mundo. We are going to turn you into surgeon extraordinaire by the time we we're done with you. Just watch your fingers now."

With the speed of a sewing machine on steroids, Bernard and Rick rapid-fired dozens of staples into the middle of the lung, then like a Thanksgiving turkey, cleanly carved away the irreversibly damaged portion of lung.

Like two of the Seven Dwarfs, they whistled as they worked— today's musical choice on the boombox in the corner of the cramped OR was the Eagles' "Hotel California."

I was afraid to ask Rick what he thought the name of the song was. "Go Tell It, California" was my best guess.

The patient might not have the wind he used to while running, but at least he'd live to run again. And within the week, he'd be able to check out and leave.

When we left the OR, the war was still going on. Word filtered in that a convoy had been hit by a series of roadside bombs. Details were sketchy, we could be getting anywhere from zero to five casualties. They'd let us know.

I walked the fifteen steps into the ER and plopped down with a couple of the medics, shooting the breeze about everything from whether baseball was a dying sport to the hidden philosophies of a rapper named Lupe Fiasco. I didn't know who or what a Lupe Fiasco was, but the medics seemed to know everything from his favorite food to his shoe size.

As we chatted, I subtly examined their faces. When confronted with the spurting blood and moans of a trauma case, they seemed old. Not older. Old. Now, in a quieter time, they looked young enough to be thinking about going to the high school prom. I wondered what they would be like when they finally went home, away from the day-to-day companionship of those who understood what they went through each day of their deployment through hell. And how their old friends back home probably wouldn't recognize, let alone relate to, them. I hoped it wouldn't be a fiasco.

Wild Bill Stanton wandered into the room.

"Dude, sounds like a game of catch is out for the day."

"Looks that way, but let's see what this case is. Maybe we can sneak out later and unleash some wild throws," I answered, hoping to do something *normal*.

It wasn't to be.

The next hour was like going to bed and having a nightmare erupt as soon as your head hit the pillow. And no matter how hard you tried, you couldn't wake up. Then you realized it wasn't a dream, you were actually living the nightmare.

The follow-up call on the radio seemed innocent, the metallic voice telling us we had a single soldier being flown in. He was awake and alert, though in a lot of pain from his vehicle being blown into the air. Blood pressure a little low, but stable. All seemingly routine. One minute from landing, this young talkative soldier suddenly went quiet and suffered a cardiac arrest. It happened so fast there wasn't time for another radio call. The pilots jacked the rotors and made an acrobatic landing as our medics stood waiting on the landing pad, trying to decipher the meaning of the abnormally steep bank, crazy descent, and skidding stop.

Inside, we stood waiting, expecting urgency but not emergency.

The double metal doors made a sharp bang as they burst open and struck the side walls of the room. In an instant, we were transported to the trauma *Twilight Zone*—time quickened and people's movements became blurred with speed. Yet I was still able to hear the ticking of the wall clock and clear single sentences spoken from across a chaotic room. I could even distinctly make out the sound of squealing wheels of the stretcher as it raced toward Alpha bay. The soldier on board was pure white. Yet not a drop of blood to be seen. Little specks of dirt and grass on the front of his uniform, that was all. And no pulse.

The medics frantically performed CPR as they ran alongside the stretcher. IVs were started, medicines administered, a yell for blood creased the air. There was a hint of heart activity on the monitor but still not strong enough for a pulse to be felt. Sharp commands of "Clear" were shouted as the paddles were applied to his chest. One shock. Two shocks. Then a third. A quick pause as rapid exams were done to search for some hidden clue to what caused this soldier's heart to abruptly crash. There simply wasn't time to use special scanners or X-rays—it was all gut feeling and experience to figure out why this young man was dying—and there were only seconds to get it right.

The mournful answer came quickly.

With many explosions, the problem is often what you cannot see. The pressure waves from those blasts don't always leave a mark on the outside, but can shatter bones and rupture organs on the inside. And that clearly was the case with this young soldier. As the staff rolled him on his side to examine his back, only the upper half of his body moved; his legs and feet remained pointed at the ceiling. The force of the blast had shattered his pelvis, and his spine disconnected from his legs. It was always a fatal injury.

We lost him.

You never wanted to call it quits. No one wants to be the first to say, or even think aloud, "I think we're done." Yet, quietly, the dreaded question finally entered the trauma bay: "Does everyone agree we can't do any more?"

It was the worst question with the worst answer. But we never stopped until all agreed. It was a rule of respect for everyone present who had worked to save this life. The answers came with curt bobs of the head and barely decipherable murmurs.

Yes. It's time.

The soldier was gently cleaned and all signs of the medical trauma we inflicted were repaired. He was redressed in his uniform. The staff lined up and stood at attention as the soldier was wheeled out of the emergency room. The last time we would ever see this soldier was during this "Walk of Honor."

Some tears flowed. Others stood with concrete faces. His unit was outside waiting for word of his condition. It was tough telling them that we did all we could but it still wasn't enough. We felt like failures as we watched their shoulders sag and lips get bitten. This unit had already suffered too many losses during the Surge—now came one more.

One soldier stepped forward, shook our hands, and murmured thanks. Then he and his buddies wandered off to let it all sink in. There would be an empty cot in their barracks that night. Loved ones back home would have an empty room. And countless lives would forever have a big hole that could never be filled.

The next day we got together as a group in the musty tent and beat ourselves up as we reviewed everything we had done and maybe could have done better. But in the end, though, we realized we had done everything right in a case that was destined for wrong. The angry accusations were forgiven and forgotten.

Nonetheless, the death of the young soldier hurt with a pain none of us could put into words. We are not gods. Sometimes we make mistakes. And even when we don't, we suffer because we are not able to undo the damage one human can inflict on another. Each of us would see this young man's face the rest of our lives. But his family would be the ones that missed his face the most.

The loss dominated everything we did over the next few days though we knew we had to move on without distraction. Other wounded needed us to be at the top of our game.

Bill and I eventually made our way over to a grassy field for our long-awaited game of catch. It was much-needed therapy on our own field of dreams. For brief periods, we talked about our families, our lives back home, and how we doctors were blessed to have each other, on good days and bad. The unique smell of a leather baseball glove pressed against my nose was a welcome distraction from the pain of the war.

Most of the time, there was a simple silence as we tossed the ball back and forth, lost in our own thoughts and questions. I wondered where the soldier was now. What happens after you die? How is his family doing? What about all their plans for the future? What were this kid's final thoughts as he lapsed into death?

Just thinking about it gave me a headache, but as the catch continued, my time will Bill brought serenity. It's funny how the great American invention of playing catch is so simple and pure. It made me wonder if we should have the Shiites and Sunnis pick up a ball and a mitt, and make them play catch until they decide to stop fighting. Better yet, maybe we should have all world leaders step onto the lawn of the U.N. and toss a ball around until they solve out their self-manufactured troubles.

The rhythmic "thwop . . . thwop . . . thwop" of a scuffed baseball smacking the web of a broken-in glove is without question a sound of peace. And our world could sure use a good game of catch.

15

FAMILY TIES

IN PAST WARS, the lifeline to home was prehistoric: snail-mailed letters and packages trapped by months in transit. No news wasn't necessarily good news, a lot of fingernails were gnawed to the nub as both sides waited for the postman to appear with the written words of a loved one.

We were fighting in the new millennium of war; not only did we have the latest and greatest weaponry and imagery, we had the Internet and a satellite phone system to keep us in liberal contact with the home front. In the case of the 399th, we were extra lucky: the hospital had its own phone tent with a few snail-like computers thrown in for Internet access. It was cramped, it was hot, but it was ours.

The compromise was privacy. We couldn't help but overhear who was struggling with the strain of too many absent hugs and kisses. We Reserve docs were fortunate; our deployments were a short three and a half months compared to the ungodly fifteen-month tours the rest of the hospital were trapped in. Our interminable waits for the phones and computers were all too often uncomfortable, overhearing the latest arguments over things that probably wouldn't have been arguments if the two sides were face-to-face. There were a lot of conversations top-heavy with quarrels and spats, many triggered by unspoken loneliness and worry.

As we'd sit and wait our turn for the phone, we'd bury our faces in a newspaper and make believe we didn't notice the shouting, with one side stressed over the blown-up soldiers seen that day, the other fretting over coping alone with the day-to-day troubles at home. And the younger the couple, the louder the screaming. The calls were cyclically predictable—a calm start, a raised voice, followed by a rapid escalation to a steadily increasing volume of anger and cursing. Then came a gradual easing of tensions, with softer words, and a few "I love you"s, followed by the hang-up.

If the hang-up prematurely became a phone slam-down early in the conversation—before the "I love you"—we'd always let the aggrieved party cut in line and hop back on the phone after they had a chance to go outside and walk off their anger. The rule was simple: never leave a phone call angry.

My daily phone calls went smoothly for the most part, with only a rare harsh word. My family had already been through a tough deployment back in 2004, so they knew the rules of the game, as did I. Keep it light and try to avoid pressuring either side about anything non-life-threatening.

The last time I was in Iraq, I never told them about the hours spent on the road, or the shotgun that sometimes traveled with my medical pack. They didn't hear about the rocket that landed yards away, blowing other soldiers up but missing me—until I was safe in the living room of my home. I stretched the truth constantly about where I was and what I did, but this time I knew I had to walk the straight-and-narrow road of truth; they were veterans themselves and wouldn't be fooled. But fudging wasn't necessary—this deployment was easier and my position on the danger scale was near zero.

The toughest call I had the entire deployment was with my mom early one Sunday morning. It's tough being a parent, especially when you have a son or daughter in a combat zone, and I've learned there's little difference whether the child is nineteen or fifty.

I stopped in the phone tent minutes before the start of my shift. It was still Saturday night in America, and my extended family were gathered in Wisconsin for the wedding of my niece Megan. The entire clan traveled across the country to get together for the first time in years, and I was the only one not there. I sat in the steamy tent in a rickety folding chair, speaking to each as they snuck from a rocking dance floor into a quiet closet at the banquet hall.

As I worked my way down the line of celebrating relatives, a seeping emptiness and loneliness added miles to the thousands already separating the hall from my hospital. Then, in the middle of an emotional black hole, I was rescued by a dose of the most potent of medicines: my mom's voice.

She's eighty-seven years old, and has suffered more than her share of war in her life, starting with my dad. They were married in August 1943 and he shipped out just three days later. Months were spent sitting by the window, futilely waiting for the postman to come. There was nary a word for eight excruciating months—then came two short letters, and even they were heavily censored; the first had only three words survive: Okay, love, Steve. It wasn't much, but it was at least enough for that one day. The second letter was a few sentences longer and was sent from a hospital in Naples, where he was recovering after being wounded by artillery.

Her youngest brother, Artie, was a soldier in Korea in 1950. He almost froze to death after being wounded and left for dead in some battle for a hill with no name.

Her next worry was my older brother, Steve. He was in Vietnam in 1967, the longest year of her life as a mother. Steve, like many other veterans of that war, was forgotten and unappreciated by our nation. But not by the mothers who waited for them to come home.

Then I threw her for a major loop when I joined the Army Medical Corps in 2003. She couldn't understand why I would do such a thing at my age, asking "Didn't I know better?" All I could say was that it seemed like the right thing to do.

At her age, my mom isn't as sharp as she used to be, but she knew clearly where I was, what I was doing, and had the same questions about the war as many Americans. We only talked for a few minutes; I told her I loved and missed her and she returned the sentiment, and then added how proud she was that I was taking care of young soldiers. She then handed the phone off to my sister, who told me Mom left the cramped room with a new spring to her tired steps and a peaceful calm in her eyes. I think she just needed to hear my voice telling her I was fine and I was safe.

I wiped away a few tears. The brief conversation triggered flashbacks of being a kid and my mom taking care of me: playing peek-a-boo, walking me to grade school, taking me for my driver's test, and hugging me tightly at my dad's funeral. Quick little snippets that packed a nostalgic punch. I realized, no matter what the age, sometimes a guy just needs his mom to tell him everything will be okay.

As my sister and I talked, the tent began to shake with the vibration of an incoming bird. It was time to get back to the war and take care of some other mom's child.

I hoped my eyes didn't show the redness of homesick tears. I kept my head down as I grabbed my gloves and stethoscope and headed to my position in Alpha bay.

The stretchers carried two soldiers; both had been hit by an IED and their vehicle had caught fire after the blast. One had a wafting odor of burnt meat rising from his body. Fire not only meant charred flesh, but superheated air sucked into lungs. I now had to worry about inhalation injuries along with the burns on the skin.

I leaned in closely as the medics cut away his blackened uniform.

"What's your name, buddy?"

"Antonio."

"I'm Dr. Hnida, Antonio. Where you from?"

"California, just outside of L.A. Near the beach."

"Kind of like here. Lots of sand, but I think you forgot to bring the ocean."

His mouth bent into a small, crooked grin—his teeth extra white against the smoke-stained skin of his face.

So far so good. I needed to look at the burns a little closer, but at least I knew he could talk—and if he could talk, he could breathe— and if he could breathe, his airways weren't fried shut. And a smile told me he wasn't going anywhere bad soon. He'd need some surgery to clean up his wounds and a close eye to make sure his airways didn't swell over the next several hours.

"Hey, I'm going over to your buddy. Just tell the folks if you need more pain medicine. You're going to be fine. Why don't you read some old magazines from 1972 we keep in our waiting room."

Out came a small chuckle that had to hurt the burnt flesh.

"Thanks, Doc."

"Don't thank me yet; wait until you get my bill. I get time and a half on the weekend."

I scooted around the cluster of medics starting IVs and cleaning the wounds.

Kneeling down at the next stretcher, I saw the wide eyes of a ter- rified soldier. This morning young and invincible, now scared and vulnerable.

"Hey, buddy, I'm Dr. Hnida. And me and my crew are going to get you all fixed up."

There were two rules I needed to follow when dealing with the wounded. The first was introducing myself as "Dr. Hnida." Iraq was the first place I'd ever done that, I usually wanted people to call me "Dave." But if there was one thing I learned about medical care in a combat zone, it was a wounded soldier wanted a "Doctor" to take care of them—not a "Dave," or even a "Major" for that matter.

The second rule was to make sure that one buddy always knew how the other buddy was doing. Sure, a soldier was worried about his wound, but he always seemed to fret more about the unknown injuries of a friend on the neighboring stretcher.

"Antonio is fine and says hi. So he's good. How about you?"

"Man, I hurt, especially my leg."

"It looks a little gnarly but it isn't going anywhere. We'll take a couple of X-rays and square you away. Hey, what's your name and where you from?"

"Todd. From Indiana."

"It rings a bell. In America, right?"

"Yes, sir," he chuckled. "Right smack in the middle."

"Well, Todd, you're going to be on crutches for a while but nothing is going to fall off when you walk around back home in the land of Hoosiers."

I turned to the medics after finishing my exam.

"Let's grab some films. Please give Dr. Stanton a call for Mr. Todd here and Dr. Nunnally for Mr. Antonio."

I went over and parked myself at my desk. One of the medics wandered over and told me he was the bearer of bad news. Oh damn.

"Sir, some strange goings-on around camp the last couple of days. I mean, this is all rumor, you understand. But anyway, seems Moe, Larry, and Curly had a few mishaps."

Ah, the revenge of the medics.

"Yeah, it seems Moe was sitting in a porta-john when a truck backed up against the door. Heard he was stuck for a while in the heat and stink. People walking by must have thought they were hearing things. A lot of yelling coming from the house of poop."

I didn't want to know any more details. But I certainly enjoyed the mental portrait of a screaming man stuck in 130-degree stench.

"Then Larry was taking a shower over in the trailer. Somebody must have taken his towel and clothes by mistake. Heard he had to streak back to the barracks. With that body, heard it was ugly. PTSD ugly."

That was a picture I didn't want to see.

"Then the air conditioner ghost came by the barracks. You know, the one who plays with the air-conditioning fuse box. Flips a switch. Turns it off. Guy comes out of his sizzling-hot room only to hear the air start running again when the fuse is flipped back on. Man, when that happens fifteen, twenty times, gotta be aggravating. That ghost sure must have been mad at Curly."

And so were a lot of other people—for a long time. It seemed this trio of administrators had a knack for dishing out platters of grief instead of support. Our group of doctors caught our share of crap but it was minimal compared to what the staff endured. The worst came the day the young American died in our ER. The three went solemn, seeking out and consoling the guys in the dead soldier's unit, as they should. But they said nothing to assuage the ER crew, surgeons, and support staff—and in some ways insinuated the death was a failure on our part. I learned it was a year-long pattern—the staff felt they were flyspecks who didn't matter in the eyes of those in charge. The three administrators, they said, sucked up the glory of the hospital's many successes, and faulted all others for its few failures.

The story of the medics' revenge made my day fly by. Over the course of several hours my patients were surgically cared for and my shift ended with a whimper. It was one of my slowest days since arriving.

I grabbed my pistol from the lockbox and decided to stop in the phone tent before chow.

The small tent was packed with people calling home on a Sunday night to America, where it would only be Sunday morning. Everyone tried to make their calls before families headed off to church.

After a few seconds of indecision, I scribbled my name on the wait list and plopped into a chair. My eyes jumped between the latest issue of *Stars and Stripes* and the faces of the callers. I guess we all must have had a good day, expressions were light and the conversations airy. A pleasant Sunday was a welcome tonic.

I glanced at my watch, more than thirty minutes had ticked

away. If things didn't speed up, I'd miss my dinner. But then again, tonight's menu was the infamous steak and lobster meal. It was the dining fare the contracting conglomerate loved to brag about: *We're feeding our men and women in the field—get this—steak and lobster! We're making this war a culinary delight that will be hard to forget!*

In reality, the steak tasted like camel and the lobster was actually crab legs that had been through numerous cycles of freezing and thawing on its long crawl to Iraq. And hard to forget my ass. I doubted the vision of a pseudogourmet dinner would erase the memories of gore I'd carry home. The hell with dinner, I thought, and would later grab a stale sandwich from the ER fridge.

I finally got my turn on the phone: The wedding was great and having the whole family there was even better. And you should have seen Grandma after she talked to you, Dad. We thought she was going to throw her cane away and do a polka. How was your shift?

As I started to answer, the hand holding the phone to my ear was bumped.

"Sorry, sir."

I glanced up. It was Todd, the wounded soldier from the morning, and the bump came from one of his crutches. He was still trying to get the hang of using the awkward sticks.

"Hey, hold on a second," I said into the phone, then looked back at Todd and the nurse who had escorted him to the phone tent. Unlike other hospitals in Iraq, we didn't have cell phones that the wounded could use to quickly call home; when able they'd hobble into the communal phone tent and wait in line like the rest of us.

"You need to hop on and call home? Have you talked to your folks yet?"

He leaned against wobbly crutches and shook his head no.

"They don't know I got hurt, sir."

I looked at his nurse. "Let's let him scoot in here. And let him use my phone card."

I scribbled the code quickly on a piece of paper as I told my kids I would call back in a few minutes.

Todd sat down and we propped his now casted leg on top of a folded blanket on a rickety chair next to the phone table. I went back to my nook in the corner of the tent and tried to concentrate on the paper. Yet I couldn't help eavesdropping on Todd's reassurances to his parents that he was fine.

"Look, Dad, I wouldn't be talking to you if I was in bad shape. Tell Mom to stop crying, I'm okay."

It went like that for a solid five minutes—the back-and-forth of worry mingled with futile attempts at reassurance. I couldn't take it anymore, his parents must have been a wreck. I would be a wreck.

I slowly walked over, and then asked Todd to hand me the phone.

"Hi. You don't know me, but my name is Dr. Hnida and I'm the doctor who took care of your son today. I need you to understand something—he got a little dinged—but only a little. He will be fine. I swear. He will be fine. Do you have any questions for me?"

I listened to the strained voice of a pleading mother asking if her son will have any problems. Will he walk again? Be able to have children? Be just like he was before he left?

I looked over at Todd and winked.

"Ma'am, the only problem he will have is if he doesn't stop chasing the nurses. Otherwise, he'll be as good as new. You've got my word. Here he is."

I had talked to waiting families after surgery more times than I could remember—and always face-to-face. This was my first Iraq-to-Indiana post-op report. But it was a satisfying one. I could see the thanks in Todd's eyes as he turned back to the phone and I could sense things had calmed down on the other end of the line. It had to be the most important conversation I had in my twenty-plus years of medicine, and I don't know if I'll ever top it. The simple act wasn't anything noble, it was just part of the job.

As I went back to my chair, I turned and looked at the young sergeant. As he closed his eyes and talked, thousands of miles evaporated. It was as if the family were together once again and everyone were fine.

16

SUICIDE ISN'T PAINLESS

I WASN'T AFRAID OF the dark anymore.

It took a couple of months, but I no longer lay awake days worrying about the night to come. Yet I still dreaded working the overnight shift. True, I was finally used to being the only doctor at the hospital and felt like I could handle whatever landed on the helipad. The medics were good and if I needed help, the docs never slept through their pages and would scoot over within minutes.

It was the physical strain that had gotten to me. I just felt like shit as my body Ping-Ponged between working days, then working nights, then cycling back to days. That weird exhausted nausea likes to attack an out-of-sync body. And by the time the clock struck 3 A.M., or in Gerry-time, oh-three-hundred, I was a dead man walking. Coffee, Red Bull, and ice cubes down the back of my uniform worked for a while, but eventually I was looking for paper clips to keep my eyelids open. Even then, in due course I'd surrender and lie down in Delta bay and close the curtains around me.

The night medics were always bright-eyed awake in the wee hours. Since they didn't do shift work, they clattered and clanged around the ER as if it were high noon. Even the movies they watched when business was slow were set on a volume that could be heard in downtown Tikrit.

But after a while, I could even snooze through that. The running joke was I could sleep through a bomb, which evolved from an explosion that shook the camp one night and brought dust and debris floating down from the ceiling into my wide-open snoring mouth. Never budged—I simply thought it was an industrial-strength case of cotton mouth. The only true wake-up potion was a patient. On this night, the alarm clock was named "Fook Yoo."

I had just dozed off when we heard a werewolflike howling from the parking lot.

"Fook yoo . . . Fook yoo."

Jumping off the stretcher, I shot a "What the hell?" look at the medics as they scrambled toward the door. "Fook yoo" came the cry in the otherwise dead night air as we swung the doors open.

The howling was now accompanied by a screech of metal on gravel. Like a car taking a curve too fast, a wheelchair was half tipped on its side as it was half pulled and half dragged to the ER. Its occupant was a vomit-covered, upside-down soldier whose head was between the footrests and legs were dangling askew up over the handles. It took four soldiers to get him to the door.

"What's your name, son?" asked Captain Thorbahn, our night shift chief nurse.

"Fook yoo," came the inverted reply.

"Hey, pal. We can't help you if you don't talk to us."

"Fook yoooooooo."

From name to unit to "What's wrong," each question brought the same reply:

"Fook yooooo."

A tall sergeant with a puke-stained uniform handed me a clear plastic bag.

"Sorry, sir, he's one of ours. His hooch mate found him gorked out with all of this shit around him."

I brought the large Baggie over to a metal surgical table. Inside were a variety of pink and yellow pills, some sugary powder, and a plastic water bottle of clear liquid. The powder was in its own mini-bag—on it was a Magic Marker–drawn smiley face and the words: "Take it if you dare!!!"

Folded into a small square was a frayed piece of paper that read: "Enuf is enuf!!! Fuk you world. I can't take this shit no more!!"

One of the medics opened the half-filled water bottle and took a whiff. His head spun away: "Jesus! I think this guy chugged rubbing alcohol!"

His statement was met with a bile-filled retch, and a gurgled "Fook yooo."

Shit, this kid was going to choke on his own vomit. We needed to get a couple of IVs in him, a few vials of blood, as well as some urine to run a rapid drug screen. But it didn't seem like the type of situation where he would stand quietly and volunteer a pee sample into a plastic cup.

"Get him on a stretcher," I said.

It took six of us to pry him out of the wheelchair and get him onto the stretcher; a few of us remained sprawled across his body to keep him from wiggling off.

"Sir, there's no way we're going to get blood or IVs with him fighting like this. He's going to bite one of us."

"Got shackles?"

"Looking for them now."

"Get me Anesthesia. We're going to put him down. But I don't want to hit him with anything until we've got an airway in place. Rubbing alcohol is nasty shit, makes you crazy one second, and gives you seizures the next."

"Right, sir. And who knows what the rest of this stuff is."

But his next move wasn't a seizure. Fook Yoo abruptly turned blue and went limp.

Some frantic words came from the head of the stretcher.

"We've still got a pulse but it's weak."

Now I was starting to sweat.

"Give me a tube. Get a line in him. Catheterize him. Cardiac monitor. The works."

As I maneuvered the airway into his windpipe, I must have hit a wake-up switch. The blue kid was no longer blue and quiet—he was beet red, thrashing, and trying to bite my fingers off. I quickly pulled the tube from his throat.

"Let me die! Fook yooo." The words trailed off like they were falling off a cliff.

Captain Thorbahn stepped up and said, "I hate to do this stuff"— then gave a "Vulcan Pinch" to the base of the neck. The thrashing and biting stopped in an instant. It was like watching *Star Trek*.

The limp effect lasted well over a minute, and when Fook Yoo woke up, he quickly got a repeat dose of the Pinch. Bam. Squeeze. Silence. Bam. Squeeze. Silence. The cycle repeated itself for several minutes; as it did, we kept one eye on him and the other eye on any sharp instruments we were trying to stick him with.

We finally got the tube into his windpipe so he wouldn't choke on his vomit, then hit him with our own cocktail of fentanyl and Versed to keep him down. We breathed for him with a handheld Ambu bag.

Amid the medical circus, the MPs came in, glanced at our patient, looked in the bag, then turned away to talk to the guys who brought him in. Three minutes later, they walked over to me.

"He's a specialist. Twenty years old. Works in an office. Never goes outside the wire. Just got extended to fifteen months. Drinks every once in a while, but hasn't tried to off himself in the past. Roomie thinks he had a fight with his girlfriend."

It seemed like drugs, depression, and boredom made up the perfect recipe for a disaster waiting to happen in a war zone. And we had to deal with these situations more often than we had time. It wasn't unusual to have an attempted suicide on one stretcher, with blown-up guys on the gurneys next to him. A couple of the attempts were guys who cracked under the strain of invisible IEDs and ghostlike insurgents. Yet they seemed, at least where we worked, to be more the exception than the rule. Many of the attempts we saw were support staff; they never left the base and never saw the face of the enemy. Their tours were twelve to fifteen months of paperwork, overbearing superiors, or problems on the home front. Fook Yoo was a poster child for suicide in Iraq.

When we finally got him settled in for the rest of the night, we collapsed in a group heap. It was physically exhausting fighting to keep alive a kid who wanted to die, the mental exhaustion even more draining. Fook Yoo would stay with us for less than a day, then be flown to Germany for a mental health evaluation.

The overwhelming stress of the night's events might have been easier to swallow had he been the only one, but through our summer the number of suicide attempts stunned us. The Smurf who came in my first days was a distant memory but should have served as a storm warning for what was to come.

Sure, there were studies and statistics—suicide rates among record highs, we heard—but we didn't look at numbers. We were too busy shining penlights into the nonresponsive eyes of unconscious kids who decided their time was up. I had seen suicides in the States, but for some reason the attempts here were much more painful. And frankly, none of us knew how to handle it. One case, in particular, I knew would haunt me forever. We called him the "Triple Threat."

Triple Threat came through the ER a month before as he was being transported from a forward base in northern Iraq to Landstuhl. We were just a stopover as he waited for a connecting flight. The day before, he'd been caught just as he was about to set the cascade of suicide in motion. His plan was elaborate and well thought out. It would take place on the roof of a building away from the hustle and bustle of the base. First, he would douse himself with gasoline and place a lighter against his fuel-soaked clothes. As the flames erupted, he'd fire a bullet from his M9 into his brain. As he fell, the rope around his neck would catch, breaking his neck as his body tumbled toward the ground. His scheme was thwarted when another soldier caught sight of him wandering on the roof looking for a place to secure the rope. Now, even though Triple Threat was just passing through, he'd require medical observation until he was placed on the night flight to Germany.

We were busy that morning—a couple of roadside bombs had broken some bodies and the burn/shoot/hang guy needed to sit shackled to a stretcher until we all had a chance to catch our breath and eyeball him before signing off on the next leg of his journey.

I felt like the guy behind the butcher counter on coupon day at the supermarket, racing from customer to customer—at one point skidding, then falling hands down in a slick puddle of blood. As I snapped off my gloves and walked to rinse off my stained arms, I heard a faint whisper.

"Excuse me." Then again. "Excuse me."

I looked up. It was our Triple Threat soldier. I glanced over at my other two patients. They were stable so I figured I could spare this guy a couple of seconds.

"What can I do for you?" I asked.

He was an soldier in his early thirties, with horn-rimmed glasses and severely combed back dark hair. He sat with his head sagging toward the floor and avoided my eyes.

"Is there any way you can loosen or take these shackles off my wrists? They've been on for six hours now and I'm cramping up."

"I can't take them off. The rules are they stay on until you get to Germany. Sorry."

"Please." He looked up as he spoke. Behind his glasses were eyes that were empty of everything but sadness.

I don't know why I asked, but I had to know.

"Why you here, man?"

In a calm, rational voice, he explained how his wife had left him for another man. These days, there weren't any "Dear John" letters, they were replaced by "Dear John" e-mails or phone calls. This guy got both. She'd taken the kids. Emptied the bank account. He couldn't get home to fix things, and said his superiors wouldn't grant him emergency leave. The only way out of here was in a box.

"Say, what's your name, pal?"

"Rob."

I looked around and wondered if I was the biggest chump in the zoo.

"Okay, Rob, here's the deal. You've got to promise me you'll sit still. Not move except to stretch out your arms. Two minutes max."

"I promise."

My mind exploded with visions of a lunatic springing off of the stretcher, grabbing a guard's weapon, and gunning us all down before finishing himself off. Insane people can act and sound normal before they kill everyone. My mind raced. I shouldn't do this, couldn't do this. It was against all the rules. I felt like I was making a major mistake by freeing Triple Threat's hands. Yet, I rolled the dice.

"Okay. Two minutes. I trust you."

His eyes brightened as I motioned for one of the guards to come over.

"Do me a favor and take the wrist shackles off—let him stretch. Two minutes."

A look of "What are you, the stupidest guy in Iraq?" met my request.

"I know, I know. Just. Do. It."

The shackles came off and I went back to my other two patients. Things got so busy I didn't make it back to Rob for another half hour. But every so often, I'd glance over. He just sat quietly. As promised.

When I did get back, he gave a weak smile and said, "Did your watch break?"

"I failed telling-time class in medical school. Couldn't remember which hand is more important—the big one or the little one."

I didn't know what else to say. Hang in there. It'll be all right. You'll work things out when you get home. You'll get the kids back. Your wife, too. Life is worth living. Rah-rah-sis-boom-bah. There was nothing I could say that wouldn't be the most hollow and worthless statement to ever exit my mouth.

I just stuck out my hand and said good luck.

"Thanks. And thanks for being kind to my wrists."

"See you, man."

But I never would. Rob was reshackled and led out the door by two burly MPs. Who knew whether he would fix things up after the mental health and military justice systems got done with him. Maybe things would work out. But maybe he'd become another statistic—a vet who blows his brains out after going home. I couldn't worry about it, at least not now. The blown-up soldier in Charlie bay was starting to moan again, he needed morphine—that I could do something about. But Rob was a patient I just couldn't fix.

It was a horrible morning. One guy had lost his leg. Another had lost his soul.

17

BLURSDAY

I SAW HIM AS soon as I pulled back the blanketed opening of the OR tent. A dark night, the moon reflected off the young soldier's dirt-stained face as he stared unseeing into the distance. He looked tired as he smoked a cigarette and leaned against a wall that seemed to be holding him up.

"Can I help you with something?" I asked as I ripped off my surgical mask and cap.

Startled, his head jerked up.

"Uh, yes, sir. Maybe, sir. I'm looking for some buddies. People inside told me they were in getting surgery."

It took a second to add things up.

"Your buddies, did they hit an IED this morning?"

"That's right, sir. I thought we all bought it when we hit that bomb."

I stared at him for a few seconds.

"We?"

"That's right, sir. We got hit this morning doing a convoy escort."

"So you were in the vehicle. You were the fifth guy, weren't you?"

"Yes, sir. They all got hurt but I'm okay."

"Well, I'm glad you're okay," I said as I continued to stare. "Hell. We all thought you were dead."

He looked down, sighed, and then flicked his cigarette onto the ground.

"No, sir, I'm alive. At least I think I'm alive."

He paused for a few seconds, looked straight into my eyes, and then said, "It's been a helluva day, sir."

I answered softly, "It sure has, hasn't it? Tell me about yours and I'll tell you about mine."

"MAN, WHAT DAY is it?" Rick asked as I squeezed into his plywood room.

"Blursday," I responded wearily. One day just melted into the next. There were no weekdays, no weekends, no true days off.

"I swear I'm getting too old for this," Rick said as he struggled to put on his boots.

"You're too old for everything. Let me get your walker, Gramps. Carpe diem. Seize the day. Neither of us on first call. I vote for take it easy."

With those not-so-chipper greetings, Rick and I started another day in paradise. It was 6:20 A.M.

THE FOUR-VEHICLE CONVOY formed up less than a mile from our barracks. Known as gun trucks, each heavily armed Humvee was manned by five soldiers. The job for the day was routine, providing security and escort for a few tractor-trailers doing a supply run from Baghdad. Before rolling out the gate, the group performed a mandatory stop at the range and test-fired their .50 caliber machine guns. The deep staccato cracks came in bursts of four and echoed across the camp. Boom. Boom-boom-boom. Boom. Boom-boom-boom. Weapons ready, the group left the security blanket of the base.

THE BIG SCREEN TV blared throughout the chow hall as we choked down make-believe eggs and tubes of fat masquerading as sausage. Some talking head on Fox News was shouting that our borders were full of holes and we were being overrun by illegal immigrants. His solution, from the comfort of a TV studio, was to send in the Army. Our group didn't want to hear it.

"Turn that shit off. How about some sports or something?"

"It's all Rumsfeld's fault. We don't even have enough troops here. Jesus, we just can't pull out early."

"Tell you what, Rumsfeld's father should have pulled out early."

"No shit. Let's go, gang, rounds start at seven."

THE GUN TRUCKS sped down MSR Tampa, the main supply route that passed the outskirts of the base. Eyes were peeled for any debris in the road or the outline of a freshly dug and hastily filled hole that might conceal a newly planted IED. A few soldiers munched on cold remnants of their MRE breakfast. There was little small talk among the five men in the Humvee at the head of the pack; their vehicle was the one at highest risk. Bob was a twenty-five-year-old from a small town in the Midwest who nervously fingered a good-luck leather wristband as he drove. Jeremy, the vehicle commander, was tempted to flip off his goggles, which were tight and blurred his vision, as he surveyed the landscape. He would yell at his men if any of them took theirs off. The goggles stayed in place.

"SO, WHO IS our final hospital resident worth discussing?" Colonel Quick glanced over his glasses at Bernard.

"Sir, it's our Iraqi policeman, Mr. Abbai. Wounds clean. Chest tube was pulled two days ago. He's ready to go this morning."

"Excellent. So what's that make our census? Zero. Excellent again. Let's keep it that way. An empty hospital is a good hospital."

AT 0815, THE Humvees rendezvoused with the supply trucks traveling up from the south. Each vehicle lined up in its appropriate place as the baton of protection was handed from one escort group to the next. The train of vehicles took off, speeding up the road to avoid becoming a target, yet driving slowly enough for eyes to scan the road for IEDs. Trash and garbage along the roadside flew into the air as the trucks rolled by. An easy run so far.

AFTER ROUNDS, I decided to blow a few minutes in the ER.

"Hey, Mike, I hear you've got the medic lecture this morning. What's the topic du jour?"

"Cutting health care costs. How we can save money if more people had primary care docs. How about you, Dave?"

"I'm up Friday. Spermodynamics. How to make your sperm work like nuclear-tipped cruise missiles."

"I'm not sure that's what Colonel Quick had in mind when he told us to teach the medics."

"These are special medics. They're real hungry for real-world knowledge. I'm even thinking of opening a chain of franchises when we get home. "Super Sperm." If you're interested, I bet it would sell big-time in St. Louis."

IT LOOKED LIKE the dead body of a small dog, a favorite hiding place for insurgents to pack full of explosives. And it was perfectly placed in the middle of the roadway. Bob hit the brakes and jerked the wheel toward the side of the road. Time to radio for demolition experts to investigate and detonate the suspicious carcass before continuing down the road. Just as Jeremy lifted the microphone to his mouth, the tractor-trailer following their Humvee drove straight over the dog.

I CHUCKLED AT the look on Mike's face, and then looked around the room. The elongated ER was quiet, a word that can be *thought* but never *said* aloud. In every single dictionary and reference book in the department's mini-library, the word "quiet" was crossed out. I lifted a bottle of chilled water from the ER's mini-fridge and tipped it toward Mike. "Here's to an easy day, man."

THERE WASN'T TIME to duck or cover heads, the Humvee crew could only hold on tight as the truck rolled over the dead dog. And kept going. The now flattened carcass didn't contain any hidden bombs or explosives. It was simply a wild dog that was probably hit by some car and lay where it had died. The crew swallowed hard as Jeremy told Bob to roll out and catch up, but not before spitting out a torrent of curses at the driver of the tractor-trailer, who had his head up his ass.

I TOOK A giant swig from the bottle and immediately spit a mouthful onto the floor. Pure plastic. Huge pallets of water were stored around the base where they'd sit for weeks in the 130-plus-degree temperatures. The plastic from the bottle leached into the overheated water, where it silently sat waiting for an unsuspecting mouth. Two of three bottles tasted like a perverse commercial for plastic and got tossed into the trashcan. We would win the war but die of plastic water bottle poisoning.

* * *

THE TRAILERS MAINTAINED a steady pace while the Humvees buzzed about like bees. The key to living until tomorrow was looking for changes today. Something that wasn't there yesterday. The dog carcass should have been obvious. More frightening were the subtle differences. And just ahead was a spot that indeed looked subtly different. Fresh dirt spread thinly just to the right of the middle of the road. The gunner stood upright through the roof of the vehicle and scanned the horizon. He was six-three and called "Tall Paul." Tall Paul saw it first. Definitely not right. Shit.

RICK WANDERED INTO the ER and saw the puddle of spit-out water at my feet. "Wet your pants again?"

After flipping him off, we decided to head over to the phone tent to check on life back home. The line for phones was short and the connections went through quickly. It was an agriculture disaster day for both of us. Prices for bales of hay in Oklahoma weren't looking good, and my lawn was turning yellow. We held the phones to our ears and silently listened to how things couldn't get much worse back home. All we could do was send each other looks of sympathy, though we both realized how stressful it was for the voices on the other end of the line. We should be home with our families, even if it was to bale hay or water the lawn.

BOB SAW IT, too. This quick jerk of the wheel probably saved a few lives yet wasn't speedy enough for a complete escape. First came a thump. A split second later the sensation of being forced underwater and all molecules of air being sucked out of lungs. A deafening loud bang quickly followed. Hundreds of pieces of hot metal ricocheted throughout the inside of the vehicle. Everyone was hit, even Tall Paul, who was blown down the turret, toppling onto the other soldiers.

* * *

"Man, it's dead this morning. How about we get a haircut?" Rick asked as we pushed our way through the opening of the phone tent into the burning air.

"Sure, why not?" I agreed. As we sauntered down the road to the local barber, we had little to say. It was too hot to talk except for a rare sentence to break up the monotony.

"These days make me crazy," Rick mumbled.

"Well, just be glad you're not checking hemorrhoids over at sick call."

"Good point."

At 0920, the interior of the vehicle was a suffocating mix of moans and smoke. Tall Paul was drenched in blood, mainly from his legs, which had been struck by a dozen shards of flying metal, as well as the blood of the men he had fallen on. As the smoke cleared, he started what's called "buddy care"—slapping pressure bandages wherever he saw or felt the warm stickiness of blood. It was one of the first lessons he learned years before at basic training.

It was only three bucks for a military cut, a simple act where an electric razor quickly buzzed over your scalp, then zigzagged the nooks behind the ears. The whole operation took a full two minutes if the barber was slow. As I waited my turn, I tried to figure which country the barbers were from; indecipherable Indian-sounding pop music blared from a cheap radio. Some Pink Floyd or Springsteen might give the joint some atmosphere. A nap was starting to sound good.

A specially trained combat medic raced from his Humvee to the damaged one a hundred yards up the road. Smoke billowed from under the vehicle for several seconds, then dissolved to nothingness. A tangle of men tumbled out. The medic quickly applied tourniquets to blood-gushing arms and legs, and started IV lines, all while trying to quiet and calm the screaming. His quick actions were automatic, but came with a price. Attached to the unit, he knew these men well. As the medic worked, the unwounded surrounded and protected him in case the IED explosion was a prelude to an ambush.

The stricken convoy radioed for help. It took less than five minutes for a pair of unarmed medevacs to spin up their rotors and launch. They sometimes traveled in twos in case one chopper went down or extra room was needed.

I HAD JUST settled in for a long morning's nap when my pager went off. *All available docs to the ER. Four urgents by litter inbound.* As I laced up my boots, Rick barged through the door. "You get paged? Sounds like they need some extra hands down at the ranch."

"I'll be ready to go as soon as I untie my laces from my fingers," I replied. "They're stuck."

"Do the wounded know you work at this place? I think I better tell the pilot to keep going to the next hospital."

NINE MINUTES LATER, the choppers landed on the road next to the convoy. Four soldiers were placed on stretchers and launched to the next stop. Bob and Tall Paul were placed into one copter; Jeremy and a new guy, whose name was forgotten in the chaos, went into the second. The men were loaded with morphine, except for the new guy, who was struggling to breathe. A sharp splinter of metal had ripped through his neck. The flight nurse started treatment in the bouncing, cramped cabin of the medevac while the chopper radioed the CSH with an update. The pilots zipped through hazy skies, trading comfort for speed. The entire crew had to make all the right decisions in the worst of conditions. The margin for error was zero.

Our walk to the hospital was brisk and we hit the door just in time to feel the vibration of blades beating the air. We checked inside to find where we were needed most. Mike was working Alpha bay, I went to Bravo, Gerry to Charlie. Rick waited with the other surgeons until we sorted things out.

THE FLIGHT TO the CSH took just under nine minutes. We were designated as "level-three care," a hospital equipped to perform more advanced emergency and surgical care. Sounds impressive, but we really could only offer fast-food medicine: get 'em in, get 'em out. We kicked into action as our medics raced to the helipad and returned blood-soaked and heaving for air, asking where to take each stretcher. Yet they had already made the decisions, bringing the soldiers in the order they thought was right: "The worst comes first." As usual, they were on the money.

"We've got a penetrating neck wound. Respiratory distress en route. Resuscitated. Vitals now stable." The New Guy.

"Multiple lacerations. Suspected multiple fractures. Open fracture left wrist." Bob.

"Blunt trauma to head. Multiple shrapnel wounds to face." Jeremy.

"Multiple lacerations and fragment wounds lower extremities. Vitals stable." Tall Paul.

We split up and got to work stemming the flow of blood, inserting tubes and IV lines, and pumping in blood. The New Guy made us the most nervous and we decided it was smart to speed-roll his stretcher into surgery before he tanked.

As Bob lay quietly, the medics cut off his good-luck bracelet. His wrist was broken and a small splinter of bone poked through the skin. A few burns scorched his hands and legs.

Jeremy had raccoon eyes, his face blackened with soot and peppered with shrapnel except for two circular areas around his eyes. Leaving those goggles on meant he would leave the war with his vision.

Tall Paul needed almost a dozen metal fragments removed in surgery but escaped with otherwise minor dents and dings, or at least what we considered minor.

We never did the math except to calculate the order each of the four customers to our CSH would go to surgery. We were too busy to think about the missing fifth occupant of the blown-up Humvee; he was probably dead but no one seemed sure.

The surgeries took longer than we thought, but we had the luxury of time. The New Guy became more stable the longer we worked; Rick and Bernard relaxed as they meticulously explored and repaired the crowded and complex architecture inside his neck. The other men were sedated as they waited their turn on the table. By the time all were finished being poked, prodded, pulled, and splinted, it was evening, and a lifetime had passed since they had test-fired their weapons that morning. The surgeries were a success and the men would be fine.

Back home, the combat support hospitals got a lot of credit for the high survival rates in Iraq, much higher than in wars past. Here, more than 94 percent of the wounded made it home compared to the 70 percent in World War II, and the slightly better 76 percent in Korea and Vietnam. But we were not the only ones who deserved pats on the back. It was a long medical chain of care that saved a life, and like a chain letter, it had to be kept intact. It was not only bad luck to break the chain, it was deadly. And these men would survive thanks to buddies, combat medics, flight nurses, pilots, and a long line of links in the chain of care.

I was beat after spending my day off holding retractors, suctioning blood, and tying sutures. All I wanted was to dig into the sandwiches the other docs left for us to munch on as we finished. First, I wanted to check the ER and make sure the not-so-quiet day wasn't looking like a not-so-quiet night. And that's when I saw the exhausted soldier leaning against the wall.

"SO THEY'RE ALL okay, then, sir?"

"Peachy keen. Good as new. Right as rain. They'll check in to our resort for the night, but should be on their way to Germany tomorrow."

His shoulders slumped in relief and his body rattled with an involuntary shiver. "You know, sir. Maybe I should be dead. If it wasn't for them, I would be."

"How's that?"

Each minute of the day was stamped into the mystery man's mind. In clear detail, he described everything: the heat, the road, the goggles, the dog, the dirt . . . and how he had made it out of the vehicle without a scratch. The other men had shielded his body and absorbed the blast.

"Thanks, sir. Thanks for taking care of my buddies. Tell the other docs thanks, too."

"I will." I smiled at the exhausted soldier. "Say, have you eaten anything today? Looks like you've been living on cigarettes."

He sheepishly shook his head and grinned as he glanced at the mound of butts at his feet. "Yeah, it's been a long day." Pausing, he looked up at the desert moon. "Say, what day is it, anyway?"

"Blursday, my friend. Every day is Blursday."

18

THE GUNS OF AUGUST

THE FOLLOWING MORNING at breakfast, we made an executive decision: our small group of scalpel wielders was going to take the month of August off from the war. The reason for our last-minute vacation plans was an announcement on TV that the Iraqi government was calling a thirty-day time-out from running the country.

Prime Minister Nouri al-Maliki said they'd deal with the war when they came back from their little break. And it sounded like a very sincere "cross our hearts and hope to die" promise. Even Vice President Cheney said it was a "sovereign right" for the Iraqis to take a little summer hiatus. And if Cheney said so—it must be so. Maybe he invited them all on a little hunting trip during their vacation. Knock 'em off one by one.

But when we heard that the reason for the summer break, per our White House spokesperson, was that it probably was going to be too hot in August for the Iraqis to go to work, shit, we got hot ourselves.

News flash: July was hot. August would be hot. And our men and women would still go out in full combat gear and patrol the country and get hot, too. Damned hot. We wondered if the politicians on both sides of the ocean had a clue about what it's like to go out in full combat gear in 130-degree heat? One idea was to have them put on a couple of overcoats and sit in a microwave set on high for ten minutes.

The cool of the evening isn't so cool, either. One night I had a gun crew come into my emergency room at 3 A.M. They had sped off the base to help a unit under attack and were out on the road for several hours lugging weapons, crawling around, you know, doing real Army stuff. By the time everything was under control and they made it to me, I had four men and women so dehydrated they could hardly walk.

We took off their shirts—heavy with sweat—and hooked them up to IVs ASAP. One liter of fluid, then a second, then a third. They still hadn't pissed so we negotiated a fourth. They gobbled ice chips like starving animals. We put their soaking-wet shirts on a scale and the dial read ten pounds. Nine of those pounds had to be sweat. Now these soldiers didn't ask for time off when they paid us a visit. Didn't even voice a single complaint; in fact, their biggest concern was for each other.

"Take care of Jones. He needs it." Or "Check Haley. She really is dry. Fix her up first, Doc."

They got their fluids and quietly walked out the door to grab a few minutes of valuable rest before they got called out again.

As we sat spooning cereal, we pondered the question: How would a civilian deal with it if they were fine one second, then found their mangled leg lying on the other side of the car the next? Or what if they were out for a stroll when they heard a crack, felt an excruciating pain in their thigh, then got hit in the face with spurts of blood as they looked down to see what happened? We weren't dumping on the folks back home; hell, we didn't know how *we* would react. But we were awed by some soldiers who had to deal with those exact scenarios in recent days.

The shattered leg guy was, first, worried about his buddies, and second, angry he was wounded. He simply didn't want to leave his unit.

The thigh guy was also one tough fellow. Fortunately, his wound was just one bloody mess. The bullet missed all the important stuff — the arteries, veins, nerves, and bones were fine. But a half inch north, south, east, or west, and that oblong ball of ammo, no bigger than your pinkie nail, would have caused life-altering damage.

This guy was a piece of work, the kind of patient you wished every patient would be. For starters, he lay quietly on the gurney — then moved, shifted, and rolled cooperatively as we examined him. This soldier even propped himself up to adjust the X-ray plate we were trying to squeeze under his wounded leg. "Not straight enough for a good picture, is it? Hang on here. I got it." Finally, he didn't even want to go to surgery and get knocked out for the wound to be cleaned.

"Can't hurt any worse than this," he said with a teeth-gritting smile.

So a couple of shots of a local anesthetic into the deepest reaches of the leg were good enough for him.

"Save the happy gas for someone who really needs it."

War was a piñata of surprises, and the soldiers were the ones being pummeled. We hoped all those who drove around with *Support Our Troops* stickers and ribbons on their cars truly knew the type of people they were supporting.

After finishing breakfast, we went through the motions of rounds, and then took off on our separate ways.

I headed straight for the Love Shack and a nap; I was scheduled for the night shift and was dragging from the marathon surgeries of the day before. Asleep within minutes, I managed to catch a few Zzzs before my pager jolted me awake. Was it another controlled det (detonation)? Mass casualties coming in? The message simply read: *Reutlinger wants you now!*

As I raced to Paradise, I didn't see any choppers spinning on

the pad; no bustle of activity around the hospital. Something was
fishy. When I walked into the empty ER, I was met by a chorus of
"shoooshes" and fingers held to lips.

"Head to the OR, sir. Quietly."

Did that mean tiptoe or take off my boots and slink in?

"Would you mind telling me what the hell's going on?"

"The most important case we've had all year. But we had to
sneak the patient in because one of the surgical administrators said
he wouldn't let *it* in *his* OR. So we sent him off to an emergency
meeting over at HQ."

Now my head was swimming. It couldn't be a VIP, couldn't be
a regular good guy, couldn't even be a regular bad guy; we simply
didn't turn anyone away. Why would we have to sneak a patient in?
And what did they mean by "it"?

The bark gave it away.

When I pushed through the doors of the OR, my eyes spied the
secret patient: Tino the dog. He worked with a local military police
unit and while relaxing the night before, decided not only to play
with a tennis ball, but swallow it as well. Tino now had an emergency
intestinal obstruction. The man of the hour was our veterinarian in a
previous life: Dr. Reutlinger.

"It's 'bout time you showed up. I knew you'd want to watch."

Me and about twenty others, all stuffed into our miniature OR,
shoulder to shoulder, craning our necks to make sure the pooch
would be okay. Worried that the pooch would be okay.

Another vet from across the base worked with Rick; she was young,
and it was one of her first surgeries. Rick took his time, spoke slowly,
and talked the young veterinarian through each step of the surgery.
Halfway through, I realized he had done the exact same thing with
me all summer. Subtly guiding me through case after case, making
me feel like I had saved the patient, when in reality I would have gotten lost in a dark place deep in someone's abdomen. Rick was a good
man, and, more importantly, a kind one.

Twenty minutes later, it was my turn to return months of favors. A two-and-one-sixteenth-ounce slightly frayed tennis ball was successfully delivered; Tino was slowly weaned off anesthesia and he awakened with a soft whimper and a wag of the tail. Then it was time to make a beeline toward HQ and the "meeting." A few of us saw the boss striding briskly back toward the hospital, with a little steam coming out of his ears. But a lot of small talk, BS, and inane chatter delayed him enough to where Tino was out of OR number 1, placed in a truck, and returned to his worried handlers. And for weeks afterward, every time we'd see any of the administrators, we'd slip one hand behind our butts and wag it like a little doggy tail. It was the best, if not sneakiest, case of the deployment.

The canine surgery was definitely worth the lack of sleep. When 7 P.M. rolled around, I went straight to the ER, hoping for a stressless shift, but it wasn't to be.

We had a series of soldiers bent and broken by roadside bombs arrives in waves through the night. The surgeons came back to work and I spent a lot of time making sure the brains inside the blown-up soldiers weren't too jarred. The CAT scanner hummed for hours as I searched for subtle bleeds, then subtle signs of brain injury even when the scans were normal.

My worst case of the night, though, wasn't even combat-related. I had stabilized the wounded that eventually made their way to surgery and was numb from the rapid parade of full stretchers that traversed my ER. Feet up, I was glad to look down the room and see a series of empty trauma bays at 2 A.M. Then I heard a faint noise.

At first, I thought the sound was coming from the medics' movie—an irregular series of soft shuddering sobs. What tearjerker was the pick of the night? Then I realized the sound was coming from just outside the door.

"Guys, something's going on that doesn't sound good."

My boots hit the ground with a loud thump as I swung my legs off the desk. Before any of us could make it to the door, it swung open, and standing in shadows was the outline of a female soldier straining to hold up what looked like a week's worth of laundry under her arm. It wasn't dirty clothes, it was another female soldier. She was small, thin, and sagging toward the ground. The sobs were coming from her. We ran to her and half dragged, half pulled the quietly weeping soldier into the safety of the ER.

She was a young girl, with short-cropped brown hair. At first, I couldn't tell if her face was stained or bruised. It turned out to be a combination of the two. We got her to the closest stretcher where she collapsed into a tight ball, lying on her side. The sobbing had stopped, so had the short bursts of muscle spasms that accompanied the tears. Now she just lay in the fetal position, shivering and silent. Her mouth opened and closed rhythmically, but no sound came out. Our eyes turned to the woman who brought her in, now she was on the floor, trying to mouth a few words in between sobs.

"Some . . . guys . . . jumped her."

Shit, it was an assault. A sexual assault. Her clothes were torn, and face bruised and scratched.

Her friend tried to tell us what happened.

"She . . . was . . . on . . . her . . . way to . . . the shower." The friend also began to cry.

My mind flashed to my daughter Katie. God help me here. During my first deployment I put a pistol to the face of some asshole who was sexually harassing one of my female bodyguards. I told him I was just a stupid doctor; everyone would just say it was an accident, that doctors can't be trusted with weapons. And he'd be dead.

It's hard to explain the rage of a father whose child has been violated. Leaving the curtains around the stretcher open, I told the male medics to take care of the friend, call the MPs, get a couple of the nurses from the ICU, and then asked the two female medics on duty that night to help me out.

It took three minutes of soft gentle questions to realize there would be no replies. I stepped away, asking the females to take over.

She thought she had been in a safe place, the fifty-yard walk from barracks to shower. Fully clothed, she walked alone in the dark. Just before opening the door, three guys grabbed her from behind, threw her to the ground, and started to pummel her face and stomach. Clothes were pulled in an effort to rip them off—but they didn't tear. Instead, there was a nasty ring of torn skin in a perfect collar line around her neck where her top caught while being forced over her head. Hand over her mouth, she kicked, punched, and bit. We'd be on the lookout for a male with an infected hand over the next few days.

Rape, sexual assault, and harassment were raw wounds for me after what my daughter went through. Hearing the story I felt maniacal, wanting to stick my pistol against the attackers' heads, then realized I need to quash my own feelings and remain calm: revenge wouldn't undue tonight's damage. This young soldier's needs and well-being came first.

The MPs were good; especially a female from CID, or criminal investigations, whose job it was to deal with victims of assault. The young woman finally let me back into the bay, allowing me to look and examine her beaten body. I needed to document every little piece of evidence I found. It was tough to consider her body as "evidence." I wondered what her father would think, if she ever had the strength to tell him.

Done with our medical role, we stepped away and let law enforcement do their job. But it was so hard to watch the evolution of looks on the soldier's face. Terror, anger, sadness, a quick hint of a smile, then eyes sinking deep into darkness. The pain would never go away, even on good days. I knew that personally.

We sat and talked among ourselves about the statistics—we didn't know the rate of assault in the military compared to the real world, but the Army was doing a better job in at least attempting to acknowledge there was a problem. Then I told them about my Katie; it was painful even years later, and would be painful until my last day on this earth. It was a wrong that could never be righted.

Although the assault took place somewhere else on the base, well away from the hospital, over the next few days we were told to be extra careful as we walked, that females needed escorts every time they showered or needed to go out at night. Even the males should be on the alert, as there had been a few robberies.

What the fuck kind of place was this? I guess like any community in America—nowhere perfectly safe—no place perfectly secure. But how could we possibly be afraid of our own soldiers? I thought the enemy was on the other side of the fence. Yet from that night to the end of my deployment, every time I wandered in the dark, my pistol was unholstered and ready to use. And it wouldn't take me a second to pull it out and squeeze the trigger.

I had changed over the years, there was now a hurt, angry man deep inside who occasionally bubbled to the surface. I didn't like him, and didn't like seeing him around. Fortunately, the kind person who lived with him kept the angry one at bay. The kind man was the one I liked living with.

19

THE WOUNDED
WORE AFTERSHAVE

W E LONGED FOR a beautiful sunrise or sunset, yet on most days in the desert the sun either rose or fell like a window shade—rapidly, with little time for enjoyment. This day would be no different. When we stepped out into the swirling wind called the Tongue of Fire, we couldn't see three feet in front of us. The floodlights were still on and would remain on through most of the morning, at least. Bad dust storms, so Paradise General would be on flight condition red until the haze evaporated.

I'd been in desert sandstorms before, but few like this. I felt like I inhaled a playground of sand before we'd walked halfway to the chow hall. And my face was raw as the fine particles blistered the skin from my face and blasted their way into every crevice of my body. Rick and I didn't even bother to try to spit a few syllables; we just tucked our chins and forged onward, heads down into the wind until we eventually reached our destination. We stood for a few minutes, shaking our bodies of sand like a wet dog that has just come out of the rain. But all the gyrations in the world wouldn't get rid of the fine particles that made their way into butt cracks and groins, and every step I took for the rest of the day felt like I were wearing sandpaper underwear.

Most of the guys were already eating by the time we walked into the cavernous hall. Checking the menu we saw tonight's fare would include stir-fry along with the usual alleged beef dish, baked potatoes, and soggy salad bar. Although our meals could be as bland as wet straw, we ate better than any soldiers in history. It's true that an army travels on its stomach, and with a short three-minute walk from chow hall to hospital our stomachs couldn't complain.

As I stood in line, I eyed the group huddled together at one end of a long table, pointing fingers and slapping knees with laughter. Jokes, insults, and BS were flying like the sand on the other side of the walls. We'd been together for more than two months, and were getting along well. No one wanted to kill each other, at least not yet, and I didn't think we'd ever see the day we would. Each of us knew we were in a fix, and unconsciously recognized the only way to survive our time here was to hold each other up. Left alone, we would become the walking psychologically wounded.

Even better, we genuinely liked each other. So much so, it was time for a nickname. *M*A*S*H* had the Pros from Dover; we had to become the pros from *somewhere*. The eight of us were reservists from all over the country with little in common except for one locale: Newark, New Jersey. Rick Reutlinger once worked in Newark. Bernard Harrison had done his residency in Newark. Ian had flown through Newark. I grew up just outside Newark. And the rest had at least heard of Newark. So Newark it was.

That morning the Pros were hammering at each other over the latest trivia—it was a double bonus round:

Where are Panama hats made?

What are the Canary Islands named after?

We had all day to ponder the questions, and hopefully we'd have time to sneak on to a computer and Google the answer.

We talked as the group left the chow hall, noticing the wind had calmed and the sky was breaking. As always, Bill and Rick stopped and checked on the guards who stood for hours in the whirling sand and intense heat, making sure they had bottles of water, Gatorade, or a couple of cookies snuck from the chow hall.

When we crossed the gravel-strewn field to the hospital, we heard the crackled sound of "Big Voice." Just like on *M*A*S*H*, there were giant loudspeakers attached to poles high above the ground: it's how we got announcements and important information. However, our Big Voice was hoarse—we couldn't understand a word coming from it. It sounded like a broken drive-through speaker at a fast-food joint.

"Vvvvepppmgrrrrrrrrrssvava. Hhhhhhhhwwwwwwchchchvavava."

We stared at the pole, then each other.

"I think either we are about to get mortared . . . or salsa lessons have been pushed back half an hour tonight."

Nonetheless, we quickened the pace, eyes and ears peeled to the sky. The only things we saw were unexpected patches of blue. That meant a day of work. It turned out to be one filled with some of the oddest cases of my war.

The first was a nineteen-year-old soldier with a cough that just wouldn't quit. Ordinarily we'd have told him to shove off and go to sick call; the ER wasn't the place for him. But something just didn't look right. A pleasant cherubic-faced kid with the weak sprouting of a grown-up mustache, his skin carried a paleness that shouted serious illness.

A chest X-ray, then a quick CAT scan of the chest gave us the reason: the huge clusters of lymph nodes signified cancer, in this case, a lymphoma.

He took the news he'd be flying to Landstuhl then the States within twenty-four hours, without much change in expression.

"Sure beats hell, doesn't it, sir? Here I am in Iraq, and I got cancer. Wait until my mom hears this one. At least I ain't going to get blown up. That'll make her happy. But Jesus, cancer?"

I'd sat and had "the talk" with dozens of patients and their families when bad news needed to be delivered, but this was a first for me. You simply don't think cancer is going to attack in a war zone. And this young man needed the same tender kid gloves any wounded soldier would get. We talked for more than an hour as we waited for the travel arrangements to be made.

As we finished, I felt the vibration of our first incoming of the day. A chopper was furiously beating the air as it hovered over the helipad. I scooted inside and quickly donned a pair of goggles and gloves. Our patient was an Iraqi soldier, and he left a trail of blood as he was wheeled in.

The flight medic told me the soldier had been in a complex IED attack—first blown up, then shot as he crawled and squirmed out of the smoking vehicle.

"He's got open wounds all four extremities, facial lacerations, and multiple puncture wounds to the torso. And double-check the groin—it's starting to seep blood. Ten milligrams of morphine on board."

Ten milligrams and still moaning, to the point no one could hear themselves think.

I asked the flight medic, "How long ago did you morphine this guy?"

"Ten mikes." That was more than enough time for some relief to kick in.

I shook my head. If there was one common denominator among Iraqis besides their ability to shoot each other by mistake or change sides overnight, their pain tolerance sucked. Paper cut to gunshot—gallons of intravenous morphine never seemed to ease their pain.

"Give him five more milligrams IV. Then let's get the translator in and figure out what we've got."

I ran through my exam—step by step as always. In the meantime, the medics performed their usual rituals of IV lines, medications, and clothes cutting.

One had just snipped away the patient's shirt and pants when he noticed an expanding stain of blood on a pair of underwear that looked unchanged for weeks.

"Hey, Dr. Hnida, this guy's got a problem down south," he said.

I mentally said, "Shit," then pulled down the underpants. The IED fragments had done a clean amputation of the left testicle and nipped part of the shaft of the penis. *No wonder he needed more morphine. There probably wasn't enough morphine in the world for this guy.* I think every male in the trauma bay unconsciously bent at the waist and went knock-kneed.

"Folks. It's gone, as in clean gone. Sorry for the thought, but double-check the clothing so a bloody ball doesn't fall out and roll across the floor."

It didn't. The testicle was nowhere to be found, and was probably still lying in some reed-filled field next to a roadway miles away. Probably to be eaten by some birds. The thought made me queasy.

"Let's pack this thing up and staunch the bleeding. Let's move, too. I'm not worried about the testicle but we've got some stat X-rays and scans to get done. Could be some other stuff happening. Look at him, he's covered with bloody polka dots."

A few minutes later, I trotted over to X-ray where our Iraqi was now lying on the table having a series of films done. Hovering over the operation was Sergeant Wolloff, the enlisted head of Radiology. He was a rough tough NCO who had no qualms speaking his mind, especially to officers he felt were getting in the way. He just threw them out of the X-ray tent. Wolloff was a quirky guy: his morning ritual included drinking coffee out of a plastic urinal while chewing on an oversized stogie as he strolled around the hospital.

"What's this sheet doing across this guy's lap?" he barked.

"He's got a wound down there. Doc wanted it covered," answered one of the X-ray techs.

"Covered, my ass. You know the rules: everything removed if we're going to get good films."

Just then, I walked into Radiology.

"I don't think I'd take that off."

"I think we do."

"No."

"Yes."

"Okay, you're the boss of this place."

Wolloff smirked, then ripped back the sheet. His face then went as white as the sheet. He stumbled to the chair and quickly crossed his legs for imaginary protection.

"Holy shit. Where's his ball?"

"I don't know. Can we leave the sheet?"

"Oh yeah, leave the sheet. Please leave the sheet."

Wolloff had seen some horrendous wounds during his time in Iraq, but had never flinched . . . until that morning. Must be a guy thing.

As for our Iraqi policeman/soldier, he did fine. And through the translator said he would gladly trade his testicle for his life anyday; he was just happy to be alive. Good perspective.

We had expected a not-so-busy day but things were hopping, and we were a little bummed—sort of like kids who think they're going to wake up to a blizzard and a day off from school, yet when the morning comes, not a flake has fallen.

But that didn't mean we couldn't have our cake and eat it, too. It was my birthday. I hadn't told anyone except maybe in passing many weeks before, but the date became imprinted in someone's mind.

One second the ER was empty, the next it was filled with marching people singing "Happy Birthday." Bill Stanton was to thank, or blame. He and a couple of nurses in the ICU had gotten some cake mix from home, stirred it up, and baked it in some little plastic play oven. Bill applied the frosting and a crooked-lettered "Happy Birthday, Dave" in Charabic on top.

It was jellylike and undercooked in places, rock-hard in others, but it was real honest-to-goodness birthday cake. And best of all, it was baked for me. We all enjoyed it, even after I held it up for a picture, and the top, icing and all, slid onto the floor. The five-second rule for picking up dropped food doesn't apply in a combat zone—I cleaned off my spilled share and ate it anyway. Even Gerry, each day becoming thinner and thinner, had a couple of pieces. All in all, a great way to celebrate the ripe age of eighty-five, which was how old I felt that particular day.

The party ended, not with a whimper, not with a bang, but with the whirling of incoming aircraft.

Up next were two guys who had been on the receiving ends of bullets. One walked in; the other rolled in via stretcher but was alert and stable.

The walker was a piece of work. He'd had his body armor off and took a glancing sniper shot to Satan—meaning a $500 tattoo of the devil on his upper back had taken the brunt of the bullet, shearing off most of Satan's pitchfork. The soldier would need a little repair work from us, then some follow-up body work down at Mr. Mohammed's House of Tattoos. We couldn't keep him still on the table, he was hyped and jumpy, I think the loss of his custom-designed devil had done a number on his head.

"Listen, buddy," I said, "you know what a bullet is? It's nature's way of telling you to slow down. It might be a good idea to listen to the sounds of nature. And don't worry, your horned friend will live to fry in hell another day."

Devilman's buddy was a little quieter; he'd taken a slug to the upper thigh and was bleeding like the proverbial stuck pig. As I did my exam, something seemed weird—I just couldn't put a finger on it.

The bullet wound was deep and stuffed with some sort of a cottonlike material I'd never seen before. Then I saw the cotton had a piece of string attached so I pulled. It was a tampon. It seemed many soldiers had been buying tampons at the PX, and then bringing them out on patrol to supplement their first-aid kit. Whatever weird looks these guys must have gotten at the checkout counter, buying a box of

Tampax was well worth it. The tampon had done a great job slowing the bleeding and helped save the soldier's life.

He needed to go to the OR to have the thigh repaired, but first needed his tank topped off.

"Sorry, buddy, you're going to need a little bit of blood before we take you in to the body shop," I told him as I threw the tampon into the trash.

"Blood?"

"Yeah, blood. Like the commercial says: Blood. It does a body good."

He started to get a few tears in his eyes. I think the realization he'd been shot was finally sinking in.

I leaned over and tried to speak quietly into his ear. That's when it hit me. The weirdness. The odd thing about this guy. It was more than the tampon. It was the fact that he smelled. Really smelled. But the fragrance wafting from his body wasn't the usual unwashed sweaty nastiness—it was really nice.

"Hey, man. Don't take this the wrong way. But you smell *really* good. What do you do, put on aftershave every day?"

His mood brightened.

"Actually, cologne."

"Oh. Sorry. I'm kind of a Dial soap guy. Or use whatever samples I can rip out of magazines. What are you wearing?"

"Allure by Chanel," he answered. "It's full-bodied, but not over-powering, you know what I mean? A touch of wood and a hint of spice. About forty bucks for a small bottle and worth every drop."

I wrinkled my nose as I unconsciously sniffed my stained armpit.

"So tell me, do you usually go out on patrol smelling like a holi-day in Paris?"

"Well, man, I mean, sir, it's like this. I'm just one small piece of a big machine. I can smell bad and look like shit just like everybody else, or I can be my own man by dressing up. And since I can't dress up, I'm going to smell good. Plus, if I get killed, I'm going down with style."

It was like talking to a different human. For the next ten minutes, I got schooled on the latest in style and grooming from a twentysome-thing fashionista. By the time we were done chatting, I realized I'd never be a poster boy for classy. The units of blood were in, and the Army's fashion plate was calm. He wound up doing great, and looked great while doing it.

The docs ended the day the same way we started it, gathered around the table, pushing food around plates, and seeing if salad dressing on potatoes would fool the palate. It did, a little.

Like a family supper, the meal essentially revolved around ques-tions like: "And how was your day, honey?" Or: "Did anything inter-esting happen at the hospital today?"

The answers were flat and quick—and normal for our typical day.

"Ah, not much. Kid who shouldn't have cancer has cancer. Cou-ple of guys got shot. Iraqi dude had his nut shot off. The usual."

We even joked about a blood drive we had a week before. An insurgent was bleeding to death on the operating table and the blood bank had run dry, so we called for all the blood donors we could get. Our soldiers responded and filled up our bleeding insurgent with dozens of units of All-American blood. So many units, we wondered if the insurgent woke up with an unexplained and insatiable appetite for mocha cappuccinos, fast food, and NASCAR.

Our meal took a full two hours; none of us ever spent that kind of time at the dinner table at home. The typical stateside doctor inhaled a full meal in less than a minute, a bad habit left over from the days of internship. A few guys gradually filtered out, but not before we covered our important questions of the day—the trivia. None of us had Google time so we were at the mercy of the trivia panel for the answers.

First the Canary Islands. I thought it was named after a bunch of birds in a cage; instead it came from the Latin *Insula Canaria*: packs of wild, fierce dogs.

0 for 1.

Next. Where do Panama hats come from? Answer: Ecuador. The name comes from the fact that many of the hats were stolen from ships as they passed through a shipping point in Panama on their way to points in the Orient.

0 for 2.

But at least my deployment wouldn't be a big fat zero—I would go home saying that I learned something, no matter how useless.

It had been a wonderful birthday. I went over to the phone tent to call my family, and we agreed I would call again in the morning, when it would be my actual birthday back home. And would save any celebration until I got home. After I hung up, I shot a quick e-mail to my coworkers in Denver. The day before, they had sent a huge box of goodies. It was already empty, quickly devoured by a lot of people who needed a goodie to get through their day. My personal goodie was the thick stack of letters and cards tucked in the corner of the box. In my e-mail, I wrote:

so there's this war movie cliché where a soldier gets mail and lies on his bunk reading and re-reading his letters. Well, it's not so much of a cliché. I spent last night reading your cards--and then reading them again- then again. Your care package arrived and it couldn't have come at a better time. We had our busiest day yet yesterday- gunshot wounds and ieds galore. The look on the troops' faces as they got to dig into boxes of goodies was something we will never forget. It sucks being far from home. Then to get even a small taste of it gives you a few mental minutes away from this hellhole. Your gifts were shared with literally dozens of soldiers--- and as of this a.m.--are all gone. You guys made a lot of people very happy. I can't thank you enough. Personally, the cards were a giant pick me up- i walked out of the hospital at 10pm dragging my butt to my bed- then took my time savoring each and every card in the box. I was up until 2am reading them and it was the first night in a while i didn't have bad dreams. A blessing since today I needed all of the strength I could get- I know it helped me help others. Now it's time to hopefully get another peaceful night's sleep. I will read your cards once again before turning off the light. I will never be able to thank you enough.

Dave.

20

TALE OF TWO BROTHERS

IT WAS AN easy August morning. I finally had a day off to gather up laundry and sweep out the three inches of dust camped on our floor. First, though, I needed to grab a bite and head over to see how the hospital was agreeing with our customers. Before saying goodbye to my room and the pinups on the wall, I X'd out another day on the calendar—we'd be winging home in a few weeks. But this day turned out to be a rougher one than the start promised, and it had nothing to do with Iraq.

It was odd how we were able to cope with the sights and screams of war, yet would get sour stomachs and jitters when we were forced to confront things over which we had no control—such as events back home.

After flashing our ID cards, and being counted by the meal clicker, we were greeted in the dining hall with images from the big screen that looked like an action flick with stuntmen and special effects. But it was no movie. A bridge had tumbled into a river, swallowing dozens of cars and people. It was the I-35 span in Minneapolis, home of Bernard and his family. As we sat with our eyes glued to the TV, our breakfasts picked at, we noted Bernard wasn't with us. He was already working the phones, sitting and fretting in the phone tent for information about the who's and what's and where-was-everybody.

For Bernard, the news, at first report, was good. No loved ones or friends involved, but he was shaken nonetheless. When he walked into rounds a few minutes late, he simply leaked a weak smile from his stressed face and turned to focus on the cases of the day. We would plod on. It was ironic how it seemed everyone worried about us being in a war zone, but we returned the worry. In some ways, we felt we were almost safer in the confines of a huge base than we would have been driving the highways of home.

I knew I wasn't the only one who stared at the ceiling for hours on end fighting the war—we all did it. And the personalities we showed to others were a reflection of our personal battle plans for surviving this hellhole. I was the wise-ass; Rick the make-believe hard-ass; Billy a noble man with an intense sense of duty; Bernard cool, unflappable, and privately thoughtful. Though we got an occasional peek into each other's minds, it was only a peek—we each fought our own war, on our own terms.

Relieved that Bernard's loved ones were safe, rounds took off like a rocket, much of it spent chuckling at the story of some Iraqi soldiers guarding some governor of some province. In a bad case of "Oops," they wound up shooting each other instead of the bad guys. Maybe they needed orange safety vests that said, "Don't shoot, I'm a good guy," in large Arabic letters. It wasn't really funny, but it was better to laugh than cry at the absurdity of a gang that couldn't shoot straight.

Since we had rushed over from breakfast, we finished rounds with our trivia question of the day: what is the weight of the average human fart?

"What's average mean?"

"Who's the farter . . . or is it fartee? I mean if we've got Reutlinger here we're talking some heavy poundage."

"What are the meals the past forty-eight hours? People food or what we get here?"

"Ask Anesthesia. They're experts at passing gas."

I stood there wondering, How do you measure something like that? A plastic Baggie? And who the hell would pay to study the question? Probably the Army.

After rounds, we watched Bernard take off into privacy while Rick and I looked for a place to hide. We both had a little paperwork to clear up, then I'd head back to my room and clean while Rick looked in on his post-surgical patients.

Out of the blue, Rick blurted, "What the hell are they doing out here?"

I looked up from the charcoal-hot gravel and saw groups of medics replacing all the sandbags in front of the hospital tents. It was one hundred and twenty-five fucking degrees Fahrenheit and some clown decided scores of perfectly good sandbags needed rearranging and replacement.

The work detail crew was shirtless, and rivulets of sweat drained down their faces and chests. Several looked like they were ready to keel over and perform an Olympic face-plant. Sergeant Courage was in charge of the chain gang.

"Top of the morning, Sergeant Courage. A tad warm for yard work, wouldn't you say?" I asked.

"Fuck you . . . sir."

His tongue was hanging like a Mississippi hound dog in the dead of summer.

"Sorry, sir. Top of the morning back to you, too. Just a little assignment to keep us out of trouble."

His scowl told us what he really thought of the idea.

"It seems like we've got our green sandbags over here, and our brown ones over there, and that mismatch is keeping some people awake at night."

Holy Christ, we were in the middle of a war and someone was

worried that the sandbags don't match? Did the wounded complain as they flew in or something? *Hey, pilot, this place looks a little sketchy, let's fly until we find something a little nicer.* It was total bullshit. We needed the medics to be rested and hydrated and at the top of their game if we had casualties.

"Who's the asshole, Monsieur Courage?"

"Sorry, sir, not at liberty to say. Never speak poorly of those who outrank you."

"Need drinks?" we asked.

"A case of ice cold Bud here in our front yard would hit the spot." He pronounced it "yahd" in his thick New England accent.

"We'll see if we didn't empty the fridge last night. Say, if anyone collapses, let us know but not before the sandbags look pretty."

We wandered off, cursing the administration. They seemed to have no concept of what these youngsters did day in and day out. They pulled twelve-hour shifts caring for broken soldiers—washed the gore off their uniforms so they could finish their day pulling guard duty at the chow hall or PX—then they had to get up extra early working as a landscaping crew in desert heat. Jeez Louise.

Back at the room, I surveyed the damage of living for two weeks since the laundry was dropped off, trash emptied, and floors swept. In our rooftop locale, we had a door that opened directly to the outside, with the door made of badly cut plywood that was so ill fitting it allowed heat and sand to steadily flow in. The most important job was the air-conditioning filter—we had a small window unit, which brought the temperature down to a subarctic 90, but was better than life on the outside. Puffs of smoke rose off the foam as I beat the filter against the side of the roof. Next came the big black trash bags. They were quickly filled with weeks-old partially eaten snacks, Mike's old *New Yorker* magazines, and a sorry collection of filled piss bottles. I counted fourteen old Gatorade bottles filled with middle-of-the-night urine—about half were mine, a couple sat next to Mike's table bed, and the rest next to Ian's mattress.

When we moved in, we vowed we'd each throw out our own nocturnal pee every morning, but it never quite worked that way. The bottles seemed to multiply like uro-bunnies. So I performed an official random act of kindness, disposing of more than a dozen bacteria-laden warm jugs of piss. It may not have seemed like much of a gesture, but in our world it was considered the ultimate humanitarian mission. In one arm an overfilled bag of bottles, in the other a laundry bag filled with dirty socks and nonregulation boxer shorts imprinted with pirate skulls or polka dots, I headed downstairs praying neither bag split apart.

After I sterilized my hands, I walked over to the chow hall to meet up with Rick for lunch.

"Three-point-five ounces," he proudly proclaimed.

"What? Your brain? Your pecker?"

"Three and a half ounces. That's the weight of the average fart. I Googled it."

"Well, when I Googled 'douche bag,' I got fourteen thousand hits with your name."

"Shut up. I win. I got the answer. I get the prize."

"And that prize is what?"

His face deflated. We've never had a prize for getting a trivia question right, and he'd walk away empty-handed despite his correct answer.

"But I still haven't been stumped yet," he said, as his face split into a toothy grin.

"Great, you can go home and years from now tell your grandkids you won the trivia question contest in the war. And the clincher was a question about farts. What is Oklahoma like, anyway? Do they have paved streets, indoor toilets, or refrigerators?"

"It's a lot nicer than Colorado. At least we don't get snow every day."

Our insults were interrupted by the chirping of his pager.

Two patients inbound with lacerations of the face. Sounded simple. I decided to walk over to the hospital with him and lend a hand to the ER doctor on duty. Gerry was running the show and said he'd take Alpha bay for the worst patient; I'd take Bravo for the other. The copter landed and in came the litters, bearing surprises in the form of two Iraqi soldiers.

Man number one didn't have simple lacerations. His face was blown off.

My guy, man number two, had a flight medic straddling his chest doing CPR. Simple? Lacerations? I think what we had here was a failure to communicate . . . but considering the conditions, it was no one's fault. My God, the chopper ride in had to be chaos.

My guy was dripping blood from his mouth and nose. A tube was in his throat but I couldn't hear any breath sounds in his lungs. Pulse was a racehorse 190. Blood pressure didn't even register. He felt burning hot. His eyeballs were bulging. Where were his wounds? We started IVs, replaced the breathing tube to the lungs, and scissors slid through clothing so we could check for other wounds. I saw none.

I'm worried about the head but I can't feel anything besides some small pieces of shrapnel in the scalp. Maybe it was more than shrapnel. We put a tube into his stomach, which quickly returned a solid flow of bright red blood. We checked his temperature—107.9. Highest I'd ever seen. We packed him in ice, filling bags with cubes and stuffing them into armpits, crotch, and around arms and legs.

Less than three minutes had passed. His head on the right side started to literally get bigger, which meant he was bleeding into the brain and that blood was pushing his scalp out. He needed neurosurgery down in Balad. Stat. But a quick X-ray showed shattered bones and a thin metal fragment that probably entered through his face— all I saw there was a small red cut, the size of a BB, but that's where the metal went in. He was going to die.

Gerry's man without a face got stabilized and was ready to go. He also needed the services of the experts in Balad, specialists who could reconstruct his facial bones. But did my guy have a chance? Do we put a second bird in the air and risk a crew and medics? I talked with my nurses, my medics, and Rick, but ultimately it was my call. We stayed. He stayed. No life-saving surgery. No surgery existed that would save his life.

The best we could do was make him comfortable. But I doubted he was in pain. I wished we could ask him if there was anything to make him feel better as he died. I was helpless. We were helpless.

We CAT-scanned his head just as the other soldier left in a helicopter. The scan showed my guy had four jagged fractures of the skull with lots of bleeding within the brain. The horrific images confirmed it was a good call to keep him here and let him die in peace. I wondered if he even knew what hit him. My question was interrupted by an interpreter who was called in to help.

We learned he was an Iraqi soldier blown up by a roadside bomb. The guy who came in with him was his older brother. One is twenty-four, the other twenty-one. Two brothers who would never see each other again.

We had no powers of attorney here. No living wills. We gathered around the stretcher to figure out if there was anything we could do to save this fellow. Change our minds and fly him out? No, not with that much brain damage. He'd never survive a flight. Do brain surgery here? No, the operation would be like trying to reconstruct a smashed pumpkin. Or do we just turn off the machines and see if he dies? The worst, but best, call. We would just make sure he was comfortable as he quickly traveled the road to death.

Yet he kept ticking along. His brain was gone, his lungs needed a respirator, but his heart was young and strong. So we waited. And would wait. Until his heart gave up the fight or we needed the bed and the equipment keeping him alive. That was the call no one wanted to make.

The hours ticked into the next morning. When we returned, he was still in the bed just as we left him. Unbelievable. We did a series of neurological tests—he was brain-dead. The heart just didn't know that yet. A steady series of beeps from the cardiac monitor reminded us.

We heard there was a big offensive push by our soldiers coming up, which would spell more wounded and the need for beds. I felt nauseated thinking about the decision that needed to be made. Our doctors and surgeons had thought of every possibility to help this guy survive but we all agreed there wasn't anything that could be done. Yet no one wanted to give up the fight and turn off life support.

Then we heard a family member had been located—a relative who was an officer in the Iraqi army. He made it to the hospital by mid-afternoon. He spoke little English. And we didn't know who he actually was; he only identified himself as "kin."

I placed my right hand over my heart, slightly bowed, and said, "*Salaam alaikum.*"

May peace be upon you.

He returned the greeting. "*Alaikum salaam.*"

And upon you be peace.

Through a translator, I explained the injuries and the outlook. I prayed that the word "hopeless" was conveyed in the soft manner I would say in English. The kin's eyes were dark and very intense; I don't think the translator was necessary. He knew. He knew without words being spoken. The decision was made to slowly turn off the machines.

We closed the curtain around the bed, and left the two alone. It took about ten minutes for the young man to die. But it was a peaceful ten minutes in a solemn, respect-filled environment. I was called back from the ER to pronounce him dead. The kin and I stood for a few minutes without a word. You could see the moisture in his eyes as well as a sense of thanks for all we had done. We shook hands, tried a few words in English, and then did a traditional Arabic goodbye: hand over heart, wishing each other peace and the love of God. His final word to me was "friend."

YOU SHOOT 'EM, YOU OWN 'EM

HE COULD HAVE been a commercial for a product promising a close shave, a *really* close shave. The bullet had zinged straight through the Iraqi soldier's neck, halfway between the chin and Adam's apple. In one side and out the other. And just deep enough to split the skin and fatty tissue, but not hit anything important. A random shot fired during a raid on a suspected insurgent hideout.

He knew he was lucky—he kept on smiling, and each grin opened a second mouth. It wasn't even close to the grossest wound we had seen and a dozen or two stitches would close things up just fine. It didn't even bleed that much. The Iraqi spoke a few words of English, and when I looked across the stretcher at one of the medics and said, "What a lucky son of a bitch," the man with two mouths let out a heavily accented "Me lucky son of bitch." Then laughed.

Man, a half inch higher, lower, or deeper, and our friend would have bought the *falaha*.

Soon after, we got our next customer from the raid—another Iraqi, but this one was on the wrong side of the law. He had been hit by a few gunshots during a firefight with our troops and was also lucky to be alive. The scenario was a familiar one. As our soldiers descended on a village, this insurgent stood in the middle of the street, then slowly and methodically worked his way toward a specific building. Too slowly and methodically. It's as if he wanted our soldiers to chase and follow him inside. He was a rabbit, and his job was to get chased and lead our guys into a building brimming with booby traps. It was a trick that had been used by the insurgents for a while, but by this stage of the war, units that have been over here and have combat experience don't fall for the ruse, even in the rushed heat of battle. They nailed him before he got inside; now it was our job to repair the damage.

As I surveyed the destruction, I heard soft moaning coming from the blood-crusted lips of the insurgent. With gunshot wounds to all four extremities, he had to be hurting, but there are times when your sympathy meter just isn't set to the same level as it is for a good guy. Then, eventually, as always, the physician inside your soul kicks in and you dose the enemy with liberal amounts of morphine and use a more gentle touch to probe his wounds.

The rest of the doctors are no different. We've all seen our own people suffer at the hands of guys like this, yet we simply follow our oath and do our jobs. I think the worst we've ever done is look down at a helpless form on a stretcher and say, "Welcome to Infidel General Hospital, now we're going to save your life." Then we go to work and heal a fellow human being.

I looked up at the soldiers who chased him down—they stood at a distance and let us do our jobs but their eyes projected a blank stare. Some of it had to be fatigue, after all, they had been out in the heat chasing down people all night, but I think it was more that their eyes were a closed door to the room of emotion. Over the weeks, I'd had a chance to shoot the breeze with some of the men and women who bring in prisoners and many were frustrated. Frustrated they didn't finish the job. Frustrated to see insurgents get four-star medical care.

Frustrated at the ever-changing rules of engagement that define when they can fire their weapons. At one point, a sweat-stained soldier with bulging forehead veins told me they weren't allowed to shoot at anyone from behind even if they'd just planted an IED; you had to see the whites of their eyes before pulling the trigger. Yet this day, like all days, they just stood stoically and silent as we worked to save those who would hurt us. They are good men and women, wise beyond their years.

And with their latest delivery, we thumbed to a well-worn chapter of our medical guidebook titled *You Shoot 'Em, You Own 'Em.*

That's the unofficial name of the policy when it comes to taking care of insurgents. If we catch them doing something bad, they get popped and we become responsible for their health care. It's a rather unique plan—a form of free, universal coverage not available even in the United States. No matter their wounds, prisoners are blindfolded, cuffed, and brought to the hospital. We doubled-check them outside for explosives, and quickly but cautiously cut their clothes off. Only then are they brought into the ER and their injuries repaired. We simply can't take a chance on a suicide belt or weapons inside our hospital. And as the Surge pushed more bad guys out of Baghdad, the more insurgents our guys got to chase and wound. That was why our August census had seen a big jump in the number of patients who hated us.

We didn't know the name of my patient, which was often the case when a bad guy was dragged in. So we christened him, as we did the others, with a special surname solely for the purpose of medical records: "Unknown." This month it seemed like we'd had the whole Unknown family come through: Sammy Unknown, Mohammed Unknown, Khalaf Unknown, Ahmed Unknown, and now, Unknown Unknown. The Unknown family had been up to a lot of dirty tricks lately.

Ian and Bill would wind up taking Unknown Unknown into surgery, then he would go to the ICU to recover. He'd have guards with him twenty-four hours a day and would be kept separate from other patients, hopefully with more than a flimsy portable screen.

At times, the insurgents really didn't trust or understand us. One guy had skin grafts to repair his burnt and mangled arm, and he couldn't figure out why the newly grafted areas had a different color and texture compared to the rest of his arm. He concluded we had sewn a new arm onto his body while he was asleep in surgery. Worse, he was a Shiite and thought we had attached a Sunni arm.

When we joked a few weeks ago about how insurgents must feel after getting a few units of good ole American blood, we also wondered if they truly understood the men and women who donated that blood.

We typically kept several dozen units on hand, but one bad case and we'd go through blood like water. Frankly, it would have been easy to just hold all the life-nourishing liquid for our own troops and let the bad guys leak until the gauge said empty. But we never did. As an equal opportunity hospital, we didn't discriminate on the basis of race, color, creed, or killer. The protocol was always the same no matter who was on the table—a call went out from the OR for a "blood drive" because we had someone running on fumes. And when the call went out for a specific blood type, dozens of American soldiers with that blood type showed up to donate. We never told them who the blood was for, and they never asked. Sort of this war's version of the military's "Don't Ask, Don't Tell" policy.

When I inquired why they rolled up their sleeves to donate without knowing if they were actually saving the life of a car bomber, the answer was haunting.

"People is people, sir. We just don't want to know which people. I'll go back and take a nap figuring I just helped save an American. If it's a *hajji*, well, you doctors are going to have to live with that one, not me."

When I walked over from the ER to the ICU for a cold bottle of water, I saw the nurses working with our longest-residing guest,

Awatif. She was about forty years old going on eighty. Almost a month before, she was caught in the middle of a midnight raid—the details still aren't clear, at least to us. We didn't know if she was running an insurgent halfway house or just relaxing one evening when a group of bad guys sprinted in to hide out.

When we blew the house up, she blew up with it, going blind, deaf, and suffering severe burns over most of her body. The doctors had done all they could; it had been the nurses who kept her alive and nursed her back to health. As I walked in, Awatif was sitting upright in a chair next to her bed—two of the nurses were washing and braiding her hair. She'll never look the same as she did before the blast—for that matter, being blind she'll never know what she looks like any day the rest of her life, but the nurses cared for her and tried to pretty her up the best they could. They had to possess a deep well of humanity that helped them deal with the next hate-filled gob of spit coming from a prisoner or a quiet moan from a broken American soldier.

Dinner that night was a happier affair. Though we wouldn't say it, we were each watching the calendar fill up with X's—silently counting the days until we got on the magic flying bus to take us home. We felt bad for the ones that came before us and will leave after us—our deployments were just under 120 days—everyone else, it seemed, was getting the fifteen-month special. That's a lot of birthdays, weddings, and funerals, let alone soccer games and bedtime stories, to be AWOL from.

In a way our deployment had been divided into three phases— the first third a time of uncertainty and nerves; the middle phase a time where we became confident in ourselves and each other; then, as we reached the final third, we walked around with fingers crossed that we'd leave on a high note. No mistakes. No bad cases. Like leaving the playground or gym, you've always got to put your last shot in the hoop.

As we sat at dinner, we all noticed the empty chair.

"Is Rick back yet?" asked Bill.

The day before, Rick flew to the CSH in Balad to have the neurosurgeons look at his MRI, the one taken at the hospital at Benning after he had failed his hearing test. Rick thought the MRI had to be fine since the Army let him board the plane and partake of the honor of serving his country in time of war.

It turned out Rick was the victim of a massive screwup. After the MRI was taken, it sat on the desk of a specialist who was on a lengthy vacation. It was thirty days before he finally returned and had a chance to eyeball Rick's scan . . . and see a tumor sitting in the corner of the brain. When Rick got the news, he somehow kept his cool and had copies of the scan sent to some neurosurgical colleagues back in Oklahoma. They assured him the tumor looked benign and could wait until he got home in September. To play it safe, though, Rick decided to fly down to Balad for yet another opinion that the tumor could be safely left alone. Like nervous parents, we waited for word that our friend would be okay.

"No, not back yet," I answered. "Later tonight or in the morning. But he shot an e-mail saying the guys in Balad thought it was a lipoma. Just a benign fatty tumor that's sitting in a bad place."

I thought about how much I missed my friend. But still had to laugh at how he made me laugh.

"You know," I said, "all that shit pouring out of his ears can't be just wax, now I think it's got to be fat."

Bernard chimed in. "Anyone who says he wants to listen to Johnny Crash or the Beach Bums in the OR has to have a fat head. That's good news, though."

No question, we missed "Uncle Ricky" at the hospital, especially me. No one for me to yell at, no one to yell at me, no one to toss adolescent quips around with like we did on the rooftop the night before he left for Balad:

"Hey, look, right next to that bright star is Uranus."

"I don't see it."

"Well, bend over a mirror when you get back to the barracks."

It was like two junior-high kids dropped into the middle of war. Our conversation at the dinner table shifted from Rick.

"Big day tomorrow, though. Mike gets his board certification. Ricky better be back for that."

Besides war wounds, butt surgery was a big-ticket item this summer. It seemed like an awful lot of soldiers got hemorrhoids, some to the point they couldn't do their jobs, standing or sitting.

The high number of cases was a match made in heaven. The surgeons hated doing them, and Mike loved doing them. So they let him operate on each and every hemorrhoid or ass case that came in. So many that Mike would be fully trained to perform rectal surgery when he got back home. Tomorrow he would be awarded his graduation certificate in "Official Care of Any and All Ass Complaints," as well as being promoted from major to *rear admiral*. Too bad his wife and kids couldn't make it to the ceremony.

The final item on the dinner menu was our upcoming rooftop party: the politically incorrect "Hos and Pimps Farewell Extravaganza." The invitation was clear: the females would dress up like pimps and the men as . . . women of the evening. The swankier the better. The more bizarre the better. I decided I would go as "Helga the hooker." Rick as "Betty Boob."

After dinner, I went back to my room for a big project: mailing all my excess stuff home. Even though it would be weeks before I'd see my front door, it would take that long for a big box of junk to arrive . . . and anything I could stuff in would be less poundage to lug. I dropped in a note:

Dear guys,

I'm sending along some extra stuff I don't think I'll need the rest of my time here. A bunch of books (which I haven't read), some spare clothing, boots, and a beat-up pair of running shoes. Sorry for the smell. Take extra good care of

the Ziploc bag filled with index cards. I spent the first few
nights here scribbling crib notes on them—they were my
cheat sheets for taking care of the wounded. I carried them
everywhere I went—the good news is I never needed
them. Not even once. A couple of cards are bloody but
that's only because I used them to scribble wound locations
in people who were blown into a lot of pieces—I couldn't
recite them fast enough to the nurse, so I just looked at the
patients and wrote what I saw as I worked. Funny, I thought
I would need these cards every single day I went to work.
Never did. Put them in a safe place—they will always remind me of how scared I was when I first got here. So
when I get home and think I'm having a bad day—I'll pull
them out and get a reality check.

I needed a break, so I walked to my locker for an energy bar and
a Gatorade. As I got to the corner of my room, my body was slammed
into the open door of my metal locker. A breath later came the loudest explosion I'd ever heard. I shook the blurriness from my head and
waited for a few seconds. I was stunned that anything could make
a concrete building shake like a rag doll. I headed outside my door
onto the roof and saw that a rocket had hit yards from the building.
We'd had a safe deployment with only a smattering of mortars and
rockets—and most of those were duds. You'd be walking along, hear
a clank and a screech as a round landed on the gravel, then skidded a
few yards harmlessly to a halt.

This one, though, carried death. When it hit, the rocket left a
huge crater and set some fires. But at this point, it didn't look like
there were any casualties.

My dad told me he hated mortars and rockets more than anything, and I understood why. There wasn't a hole you could dig that
was deep enough for protection.

As I watched a group gather on the roof to watch the results of the fireworks show, I thought of the first rocket that zipped my scalp. April 2004. I was crossing a causeway over a small lake with a group of guys when we heard a big pop. Someone said, "Don't worry, that's just a mortar hitting." We yelled a collective "Bullshit" and contemplated an emergency dive into the water when the rocket whirled overhead. The pop was actually the rocket launch and we knew it had to come down somewhere. The shell missed us, but not the arms and legs of a group of people in a small building less than a hundred yards away. I could still hear their screams. Now I watched a group of gawkers on our roof looking to see if there would be an encore. But I knew the top of a building was the last place any of us should be.

We were saved by the chirping of our pagers: report to the hospital for accountability. Meaning, we didn't have wounded to treat, we just needed to all make an appearance and show them we were alive. But since the rule was all helmets and body armor was to be stored at the hospital, we'd make a fast trip across the gravel and hope another round didn't hit. Great planning. It made me beg for my old commanders from 2004, like Izzy Rommes, who really knew war.

I finished my note before I sealed the box and headed to accountability:

> Just a couple of thoughts to end up with. I really want to say I'm sorry. I joined the Army at an old age and left you behind to worry. It's been kind of hard on me sometimes—most of the soldiers I see are your ages. When they are lying on the stretchers wounded, I look in their eyes, and I often see one of you. Coming here was a good thing, as painful as it's been for all of us. Thank you for that.
>
> I don't think I've ever explained all the reasons behind my decision—you know a lot had to do with your grandfather. I wish you could have met him. A funny guy but he carried a lot of demons—sometimes I think it was my job here to lay some of those demons to rest—but you know,

they don't make shovels strong enough or holes deep enough to bury the past. Even though we can learn from the past, we just can't undo it. We can only look forward and, even then, be ready for what life throws at us. We adjust or we spend our lives in misery complaining. As the old saying goes: Get busy living or get busy dying. When I look at all of you, I see you've chosen well. Stay on that path and you will change the world. Even if that world is one person. My accomplishment here, I hope, is at least one soldier, who because of me will someday have the chance to look at today and remember it as just some rotten day in the past. And a future with unlimited horizons.

I've got something to give you, but it's better hand-carried than mailed. It's the diary from my war.

Love, Dad

22

DOG KENNELS

I F THERE WAS one thing the Iraqis were good at, it was hurting
each other.

A couple of days ago Bernard spent five hours in the OR
piecing together the face of an Iraqi policeman who was pushed off
the back of a moving truck by his fellow cops. The effect of asphalt
on a skidding face was to pull the skin and muscle off like a Hallow-
een mask. Hanging by a flap, you could lift the face directly over the
underlying bones. It was a one-man repair job, but I kept Bernard
company as he tried to make a formerly handsome guy look like a
human again. A few months ago, I would have vomited at the sight,
now I just stood and chatted with Bernard as if we were talking about
which team had the best chance to beat the Red Sox this year.

"I called Balad since the muscles around the eye are probably still
lying on the road—but they said he's not worth flying down. So here
I am, like an old grandmother, quilting away. I just don't know what
goes where." Beads of sweat were building on Bernard's face from the
painstaking work.

I told him, "Actually, it looks pretty good. But Jesus, it was his buddies that did this? I'd hate to see what they would have done if they didn't like him."

"You got that right. Say, need a ride back to the barracks later? We can sit in the back of the truck and talk about you busting my balls over Captain Dee. Just hold on tight when we drive, man."

I rubbed my still intact face and answered a quick "No, thanks."

Yet the Iraqi policeman was just a single illustration of the hatred that was part of daily life in Iraq. Frankly, he was a nonnewsworthy speck compared to the eight hundred who died in a series of bombings in Qataniyah a few days before. All told, more than eighteen hundred Iraqis would die during the month at the hands of their countrymen; who knew the number of wounded.

Surprisingly, we rarely took care of civilians wounded in car bombs—a fact that seemed to confuse a lot of people back home. After a news report on some massive bomb, I'd hear "You sure must be busy." And yeah, I was busy, but the hospital cup wasn't overflowing with civilians. Although we did take care of the Iraqi army and some Iraqi police, we only opened our helipad to civilians if they worked with us or got caught in the middle of the crossfire—like the ancient woman Awatif. When I first got here, I thought I'd be working on Iraqis all the time, especially kids, but we were told right off the bat we had a new hands-off policy for civilians. Seemed cruel at the time, but when I went to a division surgeons meeting at the 25th Infantry back in June, that directive made sense.

Think about it: our primary job was to care for American soldiers. And it was really hard to send helicopters, vehicles, or put troops at risk picking up wounded civilians from all corners of the country. As the commanding general of our medical brigade wisely said, "I run the world's biggest trauma center. I don't run a full-service hospital."

Plus, we simply didn't have the room or the staff to care for the entire country's medical needs, even when there were mass casualties. It was the ugly and harsh reality in this neck of the world. I knew it frustrated a guy like Mike, who would have liked to save the Iraqi people, but at this point I think we were just trying to save ourselves first and foremost.

There was also the issue of getting the Iraqis to step up to the plate and run their own damn country, not just the security but its medical care as well. As we tried to get them to do so, we needed to step out of the way and force them to develop a system that was appropriate for their culture. An American-style health care system would not work here. Unfortunately, the current Iraqi civilian health care system didn't work here, either. It sucked. But that wasn't from a lack of trying on our part.

One of the best examples of failure was TTH, or by its proper moniker: Tikrit Teaching Hospital, the main hospital in Saddam's hometown. The United States had sunk more than $30 million into this place for equipment and supplies. But where that $30 million went was anyone's guess. Not equipment or supplies. Probably into some guy's pockets, the universal destination of much of the funds we pumped into this country.

We called TTH and other Iraqi hospitals "dog kennels," and for good reason—there was no nursing care. Meaning your family had better be around if you needed your wounds treated, dressings changed, even your Ambu bag squeezed. The family typically set up camp next to your bed and cooked your food as well. As for rules— there were none. Smoking was allowed even with oxygen running (when there was oxygen). All those cigarettes left a layer of smoke swirling throughout the wards. Bandages were reused and hopefully you didn't get a bed stained with old, dried blood, which I suppose was better than one damp with new blood.

Beds and basinets just sat in the parking lot, empty of patients but full of dirt and sand. TTH did have a spanking-new MRI machine and CAT scanner—but they were broken and unused—the money for replacement parts privately pocketed. The emergency crash cart had empty drawers. Bugs crawled up the walls and down onto patients. Completing the picture of a hospital from hell were the layers of dirt and mud coating the floors. The only thing missing were packs of wild dogs wandering the hallways—instead, they gathered outside and scrounged for scraps of used bandages.

· And that was the bright side of the situation—the bad was a patient had better be of the correct religious sect when going to the hospital or else the trip would be a one-way journey. We all knew if a Sunni went to a Shiite hospital or if a Shiite went to a Sunni place, it was a roll of the dice whether a patient would be assaulted or killed. So when we transferred an Iraqi out of the CSH into the civilian system, we made sure they went to the right place; it was even more important than their being stable enough for transfer. Allah help any Iraqi sent to a hospital without family, friends, or the correct religious membership card. Recently forty patients from the wrong side of the religious tracks went into the hospital in Kirkuk and were dead within twenty-four hours.

At rounds each morning, no one was vaccinated from criticism from Dr. Quick, but it was the liaisons and translators that caught the most heat. They were the ones responsible for getting patients out the door and into the Iraqi system—as ugly as the system was. Quick wanted the Iraqis discharged ASAP, but to the right place. No sense sending a Sunni to Shiite General or vice versa—all you got back was a dead patient.

The issue of "where are we going to send these patients" was big at rounds this particular morning. We'd just gotten in a batch of Iraqi police from up the road at Bayjii, a small town north of Tikrit. These people were guarding something—it wasn't clear what—when they saw something suspicious and opened fire. At each other. The ER was packed with cops full of holes. We patched them up, they'd stay a few days, then be sent to the right hospital. The liaisons were already working the Iraqi grapevine for a place for these guys to recover, and family members to become instant medical experts.

In the meantime, we were still busting Bill Stanton over his bedside manner the day before, when the group first came through the doors. The ER was instant chaos—a million voices chattering over each other, the extra noise coming from the translators we needed to communicate with the Iraqis. Bill was the busiest doctor that day— he had his hands full with bone injuries—and was zipping from stretcher to stretcher, poking and prodding and trying to reassure the patients they'd be fine. The translators were good; they could listen to our rapid-fire English, convert it to Arabic, then quickly convert the response back to English. But I think for the first time in this war they got stumped. As Bill tried to talk and ask questions of a wounded Iraqi, the translator interrupted with a confused look: "Excuse me, sir, what is word: 'dude'? Is that a person or an injury?"

As we finished up rounds, a familiar face strolled in. Rick had made it home from his brain tumor consultation in Balad in one piece, sporting the wide crooked grin of a kid who had just come back from the amusement park. And in a way, he had. As he flew into camp on a Black Hawk helicopter, the bird passed over a firefight just outside our gate. The pilot looked to see if any support was needed, the chopper rocking, bobbing, and weaving as it spiraled down to avoid any rockets or gunfire. Just the kind of stuff Rick loved—we could picture him whooping and hollering as the speeding circles got tighter and the ground swooped up toward the chopper. A total nut bag.

The flight was "administrative," meaning it was a routine trans-port of noncombat personnel, so it was filled with a bunch of folks not used to the idea of getting killed by a stray RPG—rocket-propelled grenade—or strapped into a copter barreling toward the ground dur-ing a firefight. Rick said more than one guy peed his pants in ter-ror. We stared at *his* crotch. Dry as the desert. The only odd thing was his bulging pockets. I realized they were filled with Harika Tats, and when he caught me staring, Rick answered, "I never leave home without 'em."

Even better than the war story was the confirmation of his e-mail, which said his brain was okay, or at least by his standards was okay.

The neurosurgeons at Balad said the tumor could simply be observed; no need to go under the knife. He'd stay the rest of the deployment, even though we only had a couple of weeks to go.

"So how was Balad?" I asked. It was a place we called almost every day, but never knew what things looked like on the other end of the satellite phone link.

"You should see this place. A few years ago, they were just a bunch of tents, but now, holy smokes. Beautiful chow halls, an outdoor pool with lounge chairs, rock climbing wall in their gym, and an official movie theater with padded seats and popcorn."

Okay, we had a nice chow hall, but after that, we came in dead last in the beauty competition. Our swimming pool was bomb-damaged and bone-dry, the only rocks we had were the ones we stumbled over each day as we walked to work, and our movie theater was small and portable—personal computers we crowded around to watch DVDs. It was true; we had a bad case of Air Force envy.

"So did they tell you why you mumble your words and bastardize everybody's names?" I asked.

"Nope, but it's not because of the tumor. It's just me."

Which made me feel better. I wasn't mocking someone with a brain tumor, I was dealing with a medical mystery dressed as a surgeon—a guy who when looking at a badly broken arm would say, "This patient has a fraction of his radial."

"You mean fracture of the radius."

"That's what I said."

"Christ, man, we're not doing math problems with tires here. Bones. Skeleton. Hard long things inside the body filled with calcium."

"I know. Orthopedic stuff. That's why we got Stalin."

"You mean Stanton."

"That's what I said."

The thoughts of his lunacy made me laugh, and I wandered off and said a quick prayer thanking God my friend had made it back in one piece. We lived a safe life here, much different from what I found myself in a few times in '04. Under my breath, I muttered a curse at myself for putting my family through this deployment. I was okay, but every day they probably still worried I'd get wounded or killed. I knew differently, or at least talked myself into believing differently, yet I wondered if every time the TV back home blared news of "Another death in Iraq," the heartbeats in my household screeched to a halt until details spilled out. Relief on one hand, sorrow on the other. I was fine but another family would now begin a new life minus a loved one.

I stopped in the phone tent and decided to make a quick call home.

I'm doing okay, I said. No, nothing was up. Everything was fine. Just wanted to tell everyone I love them. Be home in a bit. Look for a box with some stuff. Yeah, my friends were fine. Glad the Rockies were starting to win some ball games. Talk to you soon.

The hollow click at the end of the call matched the loneliness in my heart. What the hell was I thinking coming here? It wasn't only me serving my penance; I had sentenced my loved ones to serve it as well. How could I be so selfish? I hoped one day I'd look back and believe I did the right thing, maybe helped a few people, and didn't irreparably harm others. But that day was in another dimension. I couldn't see it or feel it. I couldn't even imagine it. I needed to sleep before my final night shift.

I WAS STILL in the dumps as I slipped my holster off my belt and put it in the lockbox. I wished I could lock up my darkened mood as well.

"It's going to be a good night tonight, Dr. Hnida. Can feel it in the air," one of my medics said.

The only thing I could feel in the air were swirling hot particles of sand being blown across the compound as I walked to the hospital, followed by the running-into-a-brick-wall shock of air conditioners turned up to frigid as I opened the doors to the ER. No T-shirt tonight, I'd work in the long sleeves of my uniform top.

"Yeah, let's make it good." I paused, knowing there was only one person who could lift me out of the dumps tonight. Me.

"Feel like getting promoted tonight?" I asked.

"Why not? I'm officer material," answered my medic.

I marched over, yanked the Velcro sergeant stripes off his uniform, and traded it for the golden oak leaf of major.

"Let's get to work."

It wasn't long before the first customers of the night showed up, the first one a fellow with bites in all the wrong places. He had been out for a twilight run when he felt a pinch in his thigh. Then another pinch a little higher. Another yet higher. He finally stopped running when the next nip nailed him right in the penis.

When he screeched to a halt and pulled down his shorts, a decent-sized scorpion dropped out. By the time he got to the ER, his penis was the size of the Goodyear Blimp. And definitely more painful. The good news for him was the larger the scorpion, the less toxic the venom. The bad news was the larger the scorpion the bigger the claws. While slipping on his shorts, our runner had committed the cardinal sin of getting dressed in Iraq: he didn't shake out his clothes.

After seeing the monster penis, I vowed to shake out every single piece of clothing twice—instead of the standard once—before it went on my body.

He was followed into the ER by a guy with a kidney stone and another with a twisted ankle from a softball game. Easy-peasy. And a couple of confused looks about why an older sergeant was taking care of them, and giving orders to a baby-faced major of twenty-two. We were having a good night until the sky erupted and angrily rained wounded.

A convoy was hit by a couple of IEDs and our trauma bays went from empty to full in minutes. Before waking everybody up over in the barracks, I strode from one end of the room to the other. Nothing too serious at first glance. Everyone was conscious, alert; there was a little bit of blood but no gaping holes. And arms and legs were attached and working. It would take a while, but we could handle this without reinforcements.

One by one, I again went from stretcher to stretcher—a longer glance and a few words to each occupant to make sure everyone knew they were okay and still on planet earth. So far so good. And a roomful of men and women who had just had an unexpected appointment with an improvised explosive device.

It attacked with a bright flash that was quickly followed by a horrendous boom and pressurized blast wave that painfully smashed bodies and caused eardrums to burst. I'd tell people to imagine the loudest fireworks display they've ever heard and multiply it by ten thousand. Even when it wasn't that bad a blast, you were stunned and confused as the interior of your vehicle filled up with smoke and dust—you could faintly hear the echo of voices screaming to see if anyone was hurt. The ringing in your ears got louder as the seconds passed. You fumbled and checked your body parts. Everything hurt since you'd been shaken like a rag doll, and you hoped when you struggled out of your vehicle no one was waiting outside to shoot at you.

There was no magic number of blasts that bought you a ticket home—but we were really aggressive in making sure the soldiers were kept off duty until they were perfect, and if there was even a twinge of doubt we erred on the side of caution. Sometimes that caused a little conflict with the battle commanders—they were always short of people for missions, but once you explained the whats and whys of a blast to the head, they usually quickly backed off and put the soldiers' well-being first. I never lost a rare argument with a commander who wanted to force a soldier back into the fight.

That was for the soldiers who walked away from their vehicles after a blast. The saddest stories were about those who did not. A blast could be a very odd thing—depending on the size and location of the explosion, some guys would untouched while others sitting next to them would be killed. Often, one body would act like a shield for the others, yet no one knew when the vehicle pulled out of camp who might be the shield of the mission.

Our medics went to work doing memory and word-association tests, called MACE exams, on our five guys. I circled the room as I watched and listened. It sounded like a couple needed a CAT scan, the others just some time off. As I eavesdropped, I noticed a young sergeant enter the ER—he must have belonged to the group. He said little to us, brushing by as he checked on his soldiers.

We asked a couple of the men who the gruff guy was. NCO in charge of the group came the answer. Was supposed go out on the mission, but stayed behind. The first time he'd done that. His jaw was square and his look was mean. I didn't think he liked us.

His look got even worse as I started my part of the exams. Like a mother hen, he stared as if to make sure I treated his soldiers well. I tended to joke with the less seriously wounded—it was a prescription to put them at ease and assure them they would be all right. My dumb wisecracks came out of my doctor bag.

"A five-year-old child could fix you up. If you wait a minute, I'll go find a five-year-old child."

"Welcome to Allstate General. We're the good hands hospital. It's where the patient comes first . . . or thirtieth, depending on our mood."

"Hi, I'm Dr. Hnida, the former Sister Mary Elizabeth. That's right, I used to be a nun, but I didn't want to make a habit of it."

The patients laughed, the sergeant glared.

It took a little over three hours to clear the crew. No one needed to stay overnight; they'd just be confined to quarters and head to sick call in a day or two for a recheck.

By the time the paperwork was nearly done, the clock was striking four. As we dotted the i's and crossed the final t's, I asked a couple of the men what the hell was wrong with their sergeant—

was he always such a hard-ass? Their answers surprised me and sent
me for a walk.

I stepped outside and sucked in a deep breath of predawn air.

Sniffing a puff of smoke, I spotted the sergeant slumped against
a wall.

"Sarge, need anything?" I asked.

He looked up quickly, glanced at me, and then quickly walked
away.

"Hey. Stop right now. I need to talk to you, man."

He slowed, then stopped, hesitated a few steps forward, then
stopped again.

"Yes, sir."

I caught up.

"Hey, relax for a second. I don't bite. What's up? You've got a
major bug up your ass and I think that major is me."

There was a long pause as he stared up at the dark sky. When his
head tilted to eye level, I noticed a dirty face smeared by fresh tears
that had been hastily wiped away.

"It's not you, sir. It's me. I fucked up. One of these guys needed
experience running the show so I stayed behind screwing around in
my quarters. Then I get a call my crew hit an IED. I should have been
there."

An "I fucked up" conversation on the same sidewalk three months
ago flashed back and I shook through a momentary cold sweat.

"How'd you fuck up? Your guys are fine. And I'm sorry I was mess-
ing around in there, but they needed to know they were okay."

"I know that, sir. Appreciate it. All I'm saying is I just should have
been there. They needed me."

"Sit down, son."

We parked ourselves squarely on the sidewalk with our backs
against a concrete blast wall. The only noise was the ever-present
night wind, the only illumination the soft blinking of blue landing
lights on the helipad.

I told him the story of the first and only time I'd ever let my medics go on the road by themselves. It was back in 2004, and I was going home the next day. A little Iraqi girl had been burned in a bomb blast and was close to dying. I knelt in the middle of a road, a radio in one hand, screaming for a chopper, in the other a knife ready to cut a hole in her throat to make an airway. A chopper couldn't come, none was available, so she either would die on the pavement, or we'd have to drive her over hostile roads to the British hospital. It was a drive I'd made too many times during my tour, so with one day to go before I left for the safety of home, I let the medics go by themselves. It was a haunting mistake and I sat worrying at the gate for their return. Six hours of fretting and worry. I almost cried when I saw the convoy safe and sound, rolling back up the road to camp.

"Guilt is a horrible companion. And I never would have forgiven myself if they had been killed," I said as I finished the story.

He slowly stared up at me.

"Yes, sir. You got that right. I sat by the radio all night, then worried my way to the hospital when I heard they got hit. I was thinking all that would be left of them would be a bunch of pieces."

The night was dissolving to dawn and I could finally make out his features. The sergeant looked about twenty-four. Hell of an age to carry the weight of command and make decisions of life and death. Only a little older than my dad at Anzio. The group inside the same ages as my own kids.

"You did the right thing," I said. "Now it's time to let them know how you feel about them. Heck, they didn't do anything wrong, especially the one who commanded the mission. Don't take your guilt out on them."

He paused for several moments.

"You're right, sir."

Inside, they sat in a straight row of chairs, like school kids waiting for the teacher. Their faces a mix of worry and concern as they looked at the sergeant walking back in. As one, they stood. The sergeant drew them into a tight circle and spoke softly. I couldn't hear a word, but didn't need to. The tears and the hugs told the story and flavor of what was said.

The young sergeant was already a man, but tonight became an even better one.

23

LAST TANGO IN TIKRIT

I T WAS LIKE Christmas in summer. Only our presents came down the chimney on a C-130 instead of a sleigh. A bountiful holiday it was: a full complement of replacement doctors. And an oh-so-very-welcome group since we were all paranoid they somehow, some way, would not show up and we'd be trapped here forever. I don't think we really worried about it until the last couple of weeks of our deployment, when the walls surrounding the camp suddenly started a claustrophobic contraction. Here we were—a group of grown men penned into a shrinking half-mile-square world and now at the mercy of some faceless paper pusher who, alone, had the power to deny us parole.

It was creepy in a way. Trapped, we had absolutely no way of getting home unless the Army gave us a ride. It's not like we had cars, or could simply hop over to the local airport and book a flight home. Hell, sticking a thumb out and hitchhiking wouldn't have gotten us more than a few miles down hostile roads.

We threw high-fives and fist bumps at breakfast when informed our relief flew in during the night and were now officially on base.

We would right seat/left seat with them after they caught up on sleep. It would be a great moment when we handed over the keys to the hospital, even better when the camp was in the rearview mirror.

We had celebrated our jailbreak with the long-awaited farewell shindig: the Hos and Pimps Extravaganza. The blender was spinning a wicked brew, which those of us on duty were afraid to sample; smoky whiffs from a hookah we didn't dare breathe. The strongest substance we dared go near were the always accessible cigars—we even got Bernard to take a few puffs. He'd warned us all summer about his aversion to smoke, now after two baby puffs, he looked like he was going to launch his cookies. As we laughed at the stud-man's nausea, all he could gasp out was a weak "Bet you've never seen a black man turn green."

But we still had a blast. The party was a wild one, at least for much of the staff. They smoked, they drank, and the innovative ones had sex in newly discovered hidden corners.

Rick and I twirled on the concrete roof, giddily celebrating our upcoming departure with a nice little dance number à la Fred Astaire and Ginger Rogers. Except we couldn't agree on who would be Fred and who would be Ginger—we were lucky we didn't break each other's toes as we fought over who would lead and who would follow. I never knew a burly Oklahoman could do such expert pirouettes.

The only near casualties of the night came during the wheelchair races. A chair pusher lost his grip after running over a group of toes, then watched in horror as the occupied chair teetered at the edge of our three-story rooftop. Both pusher and pushee needed a waterfall of drinks to quell their shaking. No harm, no foul. The night was a perfect goodbye to the staff we'd grown to love.

Besides freedom, our sole wish at this point was to leave on a high note. We'd had a good couple of weeks. No lost cases. No lost sons. No lost daughters.

It wasn't to be.

Early the next morning, Sergeant David Heringes was slowly

walking around a disabled Humvee on a lonely road about fifty miles from our CSH. It was a road much different than the one he was supposed to be on that day. Heringes had planned to be in Florida, enjoying a fun-filled vacation at Disney World with his wife, children, and parents. But six weeks before, Heringes and hundreds of other soldiers in the 82nd Airborne were told to unpack their bags. Instead of heading stateside on August 1, their deployment was being extended from twelve to fifteen months; it would be October before they'd set foot on American soil and hug their loved ones.

David had told his dad to go ahead and use the tickets even though he couldn't be there; it would make him happy to know the family had a chance to get away and find distraction from their worries and fears.

So as his family was finishing a wonderful yet hollow day at the theme park often called the happiest place on earth, Heringes kept one eye on his men and used the other to scan for hidden danger. The morning was typical for an Iraq summer: baking heat, with swirling sand-filled air. Dripping with sweat, Heringes told his men to stay clear as he surveyed the disabled vehicle. As he cautiously checked for the cause of the breakdown, an insurgent hiding about a half mile away pressed some buttons on his cell phone. The sequence of numbers detonated a mortar shell buried near the vehicle.

It was a strange explosion, like many were. Most of the men in Heringes' platoon came out of the blast with little more than scratches—they were shielded and protected by one man. And that one man took the brunt of the impact. As the medevac approached, Heringes still was alive, though barely, and drifting in and out of consciousness. He told his fellow soldiers he could hear angels coming as he lay on the ground.

His wounds were severe, and blood flowed freely. Pressure dressings, hemostatic bandages, IVs—the flight medic used every tool and trick to keep him alive until he got to us. Finally, she could do no

more and simply held him and stroked his head as he quietly murmured the names of his family.

When we first heard the faint whirling of the helicopter, we still
couldn't see it, and could only pray there was hope for this young
soldier. But miles before, the rapid loss of blood translated into the
loss of his life. He fought death hard, and the medic fought with him.
Talking to him. Encouraging him. Holding him. Importantly, he
didn't die alone. And his final thoughts were of his loved ones.

Back home, we probably just would have brought him in and
closed the curtains around the stretcher. Instead, we kicked into high
gear; there was a frantic scurry of medicine performed that day. Our
chances of saving him were nonexistent, yet we had to try.

Blood was pumped into the large veins of his neck as the stretcher
sped to the OR—there had been only a brief stop in the emergency
room to get the IV lines started. In the OR, Bernard and Rick tried to
surgically repair a man who had died fifteen minutes ago.

There's often talk about how doctors try to play God, talk fre-
quently uttered with a negative tone. I don't know if our group tried
to play God or battle God this particular morning; perhaps we were
both on the same side, battling evil. Or maybe it was simply part of
a painful plan that we mortals would never understand. The soldier
had died peacefully. It was done. Close to two hours after first entering the OR, my two friends quietly stepped back from the table, and
tore off their surgical gowns. And walked way.

It was hard on everyone; no harder than it would be on his family,
but hard nonetheless. Every time a soldier dies, a small piece of us
goes with him.

Bernard stumbled back to his room, and stayed inside for such
a long time that we worried—so much so we checked on him every
few hours, seeing if he needed food, or just a friendly face. Rick and
I walked and talked for long periods, but really, it was more walking
than talking. The hospital staff went into mourning and worried, in
particular, about the flight medic who was the soldier's sole compan-

ion during the final moments of his life. She was a great flight medic, and an even better person. Whenever I saw her walk in the door with a patient, I knew that patient had been lucky, and my job would be easier. Now she was in pain. A pain that had no remedy or cure. I asked God to bless her and give her peace. And later wondered if she was one of the many angels sent to accompany David on his final journey.

I don't remember much more of the final days. The new docs followed us around, and we probably gave the same speeches and thoughts we got from Brent Smith and company when we first arrived. The day our flight was to carry us back to our loved ones was supposed to be a quiet one. We were officially relieved, and as of 0700 had turned the keys to the CSH over to the new guys. We packed and unpacked, then repeated the process again. Said a few goodbyes. Then made sure we all knew the truck to the airfield would be outside our quarters at four.

I wasn't supposed to do a speck of work that final day, I just needed to wander over to the hospital to write a couple of final reports and check on our replacements as well as say goodbye to the medics and nurses who had held my hand while I made believe I knew what I was doing. I would miss them, and sadly, worried for them. They had seen far more than I in their year of deployment, and I wondered how much mental baggage they would carry home. I was old, they were young, and would have to live with their nightmares far longer than I would.

I was scribbling away in a corner of the ER—trying to stay out of the way—when word came over the radio that four seriously wounded Iraqi soldiers were on their way. A drainage pipe under a roadway had been packed with explosives and blew their large truck ten feet in the air. When the wounded arrived, you could hear some of them moaning over the whine of the helicopter blades. This would be the first major test for our replacements and they didn't yet have the manpower on site to handle the wounded. I needed to stay.

It was a scary sixty minutes—blood everywhere—limbs pointing in every direction. In some ways, I was almost glad to hear the moans, because it meant the injured were getting enough air to moan. It was the quiet ones that scared me, and a couple were too quiet.

Most of the replacements seemed like quality guys, and they knew they were in for an experience unlike anything they'd ever had. Some eyes looked like mine the first day I showed up on the job: a mix of terror, confusion, and panic. It had taken months to evolve, but for me, this day, this mess was just another day.

During our briefings over the past few days, it was interesting to observe the mix of doctors who would replace us. Most knew they were in for a hell of a ride; they were full of questions and actually paid attention when we answered. Most importantly, they treated the staff and each other well. On the other hand, a couple of the newbies seemed a little too confident, in fact, outright cocky, talking about how they were going to do things differently, go by the book, and asking us why we didn't follow the latest protocols. Now they would be hit in the face with reality—forced to learn that pure academic or "I'm smarter than you" bullshit doesn't fly in a war zone. And protocols? Protocols, my ass. We had no choice but to make up our own protocols and realized that spaghetti-and-meatball surgery was usually the best and only surgery.

Now they had to learn to interpret things like the moans and different sounds a wounded human makes. Realize that pieces of arms and legs bent toward all points of the compass were sometimes less important than the small easy-to-ignore wound that barely made a hole in the skin, yet tore apart vital organs inside. And not freak out over gushes of blood that sprayed the room, that it was sometimes more important to observe the small drips of blood that would fall to the floor without a sound.

Of the four wounded, three made it, one did not. The force of the blast had driven metal fragments into his brain and torn away parts of both arms and legs. We did everything we could, but it wasn't enough. The new doctors learned quickly you couldn't beat death by simply practicing good medicine; there are forces at work beyond our control, forces that are very humbling. Learn that, accept that, and you will cheat death 99 percent of the time. But the 1 percent will haunt you the rest of your life.

During the cases, I did little work, mainly going from trauma bay to trauma bay, watching for landmines, potholes, and errors obvious to an experienced eye, but not to a new one. All in all, the new group did well, especially the two family docs who were jumping into the same ER quicksand I had months ago. Bathed in sweat, their baptism of fire hadn't singed them too badly—their beet red faces and stained uniforms now marked them as veterans.

As the cases finished and the wounded went to surgery, I made the rounds of the room, trying to squeeze in a few goodbyes to my medics and nurses. I had lots to say and thank-yous to give but it wasn't to be. As the staff continued to scurry about, our conversations were rushed and clipped. My day, my deployment was done. Theirs flowed on like a torrent. As they slammed and hammered, each said a rushed goodbye, a thanks, and finally the universal farewell of soldiers: "Be safe."

Then, as I turned to leave, they all added a short postscript with sly grins.

The words "See ya, Dave," "Take care, Davy," and "Great working with you, Dave-a-reeno" echoed through the ER.

It had taken months, but I had finally gotten something other than a "sir." About time.

After wrapping things up, I trudged away—drained of the little energy left after four months in this shithole. As I reached the door, one of the new guys stopped me. He asked me how things had changed over the months we were there; the answer came without much thought.

"Choppers without an appointment, human jigsaw puzzles, temperatures that make hell seem chilly. No, nothing's changed since the day I got here . . . except me."

It was time to finish packing for the trip home.

24

HERO'S WELCOME

SOMEONE WATCHING FROM a distance would have thought it was a group of overgrown kids going to the circus or an amusement park. Eight doctors shouting, laughing, and stealing hats, getting ready to board our deuce-and-a-half-ton truck for a ride to the airstrip and the first leg of our journey home. The duffel bags, which seemed so overloaded when we arrived, were tossed onto the truck as if they contained nothing but air. Some of the guys were done for good, a few of us knew we'd be back, but it didn't matter. We were all in one piece and heading home to our loved ones.

The ride to the airfield took fifteen minutes, bouncing the whole way over rough unpaved roads, goofing around and snapping pictures of each other's funniest face. It seemed like the only memories in the truck with us were the comical ones: like the look on the insurgent's face as he awoke from surgery to the sounds of Led Zeppelin blasting away in the OR, surrounded by a group of masked Americans singing "Stairway to Heaven." Then there was the porta-john tipped over by a truck while some soldier was inside sitting reading *Stars and Stripes*. He looked like a dyed-blue Easter egg as he spit and sputtered his way into the ER. Then how much would we miss the salami-and-jelly sandwiches that broke up the culinary boredom?

It wasn't until we looked at the hospital in the distance that the laughter softly died. Two medevacs with wounded were landing on the helipad. They were specks in the sky but we all knew the precious cargo on board. We were leaving the war, but the war couldn't care less. All we could do was feel guilty about leaving the twenty-year-olds behind in a war that would not have a Hollywood ending. No war ever does.

As the distance between us and the base continued to grow, we realized we would never really leave. We'd revisit this place often in the years to come, traveling back in sweat-soaked dreams on our darkest nights. I now knew what my father, and every other man and woman who has seen the horrors of war, knew: you may leave the war, but it never leaves you. The only sounds during the rest of the ride came from the thumps and bangs of the truck meeting the rough road.

We sat at the airfield for hours, occasionally herded like cattle from one building to the next, going through each stage of the out-processing procedure at the usual hurry-up-and-wait pace of the military. Our flight to Kuwait wasn't leaving until that night; we had started our check-in at five. But we didn't mind the hurry-up-and-wait; if we missed this first connection to Kuwait, there would be more than a week's delay for the next flight to the States. Admonished not to wander, our small group naturally huddled together in a protective cocoon, surrounded by a milling group of more than a hundred troops who were also ferrying out that night. Even our trips to the latrine were group events: we didn't want anyone left behind in case the Army pulled a fast one and announced the plane was suddenly leaving in less than one minute.

Outside, the only thing visible in any direction was the vast empty desert that made up much of the base. I think we were stunned at its enormousness; the hospital wasn't even visible over the horizon. It was as if we had lived the past few months on our own half-mile-square planet in the middle of a vast universe. In a compressed time, a lot of living happened on that half-mile patch, along with some dying.

Our stay in Kuwait was mercifully brief, a short coffee break compared to our last visit. Just three nights stuffed into an undersized tent filled with the smell of men who have worked too hard. We napped a lot, stood and waited in long phone lines, and told fewer jokes than we had all summer. The only prank was on the easiest of targets. As Bernard snoozed one afternoon, we stuck a piece of surgical tape on his crotch, proclaiming "Iraq's Most Famous." He wandered around in a nap-induced fog for close to an hour after awakening, wondering why everyone on the way to chow kept pointing and laughing at his groin.

The flight from Kuwait to Fort Benning also went much better than the trip over. We actually flew in a plane that wasn't held together by duct tape, and Rick and I were able to snag a couple of seats together in the back. We slept most of the way, stopping briefly for a refuel in Leipzig, Germany, where we were told we could get off the plane, stretch our legs, and legally have one beer. We awaited the stampede to the bar but were surprised to find only a few soldiers standing around sipping their single brew at 2 A.M. I guess we were all too tired and too beaten up to drown whatever emotions were stuffed deep inside.

After many hours, and several startled wake-ups to imaginary beepers going off, we landed at Benning on a early Sunday morning. A small crowd gathered to meet us while a band played patriotic songs and salutes were thrown like confetti. We awaited a couple of generals to show up and call us "heroes." Fortunately their speeches were short on words, long on patriotism, and we were herded to buses that would take us to what we hoped were patriotic barracks fit for sleep-deprived heroes.

Instead, we got shitholes worse than our makeshift plywood rooms in Iraq. Torn, bloodstained sheets and pillowcases; broken and bent blinds over cracked windows; and a warm refrigerator filled with mouse shit. The communal toilets were clogged and overflowing while the shower stalls had shit-smeared walls. We were pissed about how we were treated, but maniacally angry thinking that some of the troops we had cared for were stuck in hellholes like this. We'd heard the stories that had come out of Walter Reed in the months before we'd deployed, wounded warriors sharing beds with cockroaches. It looked like the Army still hadn't cleaned up its act.

We had busted our fucking humps keeping soldiers alive, worried ourselves through too many sleepless nights about how to keep them alive, and this is what *their* hero's welcome would be?

Rick and I spent our first few hours in Horror Hotel trying to calm each other down, finally cooling to the point where we put a sign on our door saying "Fuck the Army," locked the door, and tried to sleep off a four-month combat hangover.

All we really wanted was to go home, but before the Army took off its leash, we had to turn in equipment, get debriefed, and be screened for stress. It would take five days to complete the process—we probably could have knocked it out in one. Once again, our small group got caught up in the numbers game. We were itchy, but weren't the only ones on our way home—a lot of soldiers and even more contractors needed to de-Surge as well. So most of each day was spent exercising or simply wandering around the base—alone. After spending months eating, sleeping, and working together, we needed space from each other and, perhaps, time to process the things we'd seen. We just couldn't cold-turkey off the adrenaline injected by the CSH—the culture shock was too much for the body and mind.

I certainly wasn't ready for the abrupt rules and regulations of a stateside post. The morning after arriving, I showed up for breakfast in my official Army regulation running shorts and T-shirt after a leisurely jog. I wasn't prepared to be thrown out of the mess hall for being underdressed. I'd already gone through the line and piled high my tray with real eggs, fresh cereal, and honest-to-goodness cow's milk. Pure heaven. As the spoon met my mouth, my arm met a tap. *Excuse me, soldier, you're out of uniform and have to leave.* I was confused, if I could wear my exercise clothes to meals in Iraq, why couldn't I do it here? *Post rules, Major. No exceptions. You need to be in full uniform to enter a mess facility.* I didn't think the curses that followed originated from me—but they did. I always made a point to be courteous but ended this session with a loud "Fuck." I shouldn't have done it, but I was tired and pissed. I stormed back to my room with empty hands and an empty stomach. Yet over the course of the next hour came a series of knocks to my room—each knock accompanied by a Styrofoam container of food snuck out of the chow hall by my fellow physicians.

In many ways, the silent bearing of breakfast gifts was typical of our time at Benning. We'd pass each other in the halls of the barracks, and then just go our separate ways until it was time for some group activity. Then we'd scramble on a search mission to make sure no one missed some mandatory meeting. Even separate, we still functioned as one.

When we handed in our gear, we thanked the Army for the long underwear and stocking caps; even unworn they were nonreturnable items. Maybe they'd come in handy on some cold winter day back home, or for that matter, wind up as unpleasant reminders stuffed in the back of a closet.

We fibbed on our "post-deployment health assessments," denying we had headaches, sleep problems, or irritability. Had we seen any wounded or dead bodies? Sure we had—lots of them—but no, the sights didn't affect us mentally. We worried that a "yes" answer to the wrong question would leave us on the sidewalk, waving goodbye to everyone else allowed to get on the bus for the trip to the airport and home.

We were then told how our lives had been changed by going to war, the lecture led by people without combat patches on their sleeves. They told us not to be worried if we felt of sense of panic when in confined spaces or crowds—a warning delivered in a humid, windowless tent constructed for fifty but stuffed with two hundred.

Twenty sessions and six long days later, we were paroled from Benning and placed on a bus to the Atlanta airport, where we would finally split up and fly to our respective homes. It was a quiet journey, and at the airport, our goodbyes, at least to the casual observer, probably seemed awkward, choppy, and brief. But the thin ribbon of a smile, the squint of the eyes, and the almost imperceptible nod of a head spoke deep and thoughtful volumes. We had spent a lifetime together in just four months, and didn't need words to communicate our feelings.

We knew we would never be as close to another group of people in our lives. And no one would ever be invited to join our exclusive club of combat doctors. There simply wasn't much that could be said. Except . . . the fifteen messages I left at every paging telephone I could find, feigning a variety of female voices, all asking a handsome prude of a doctor for a final, farewell date. My memories still ring with the recurring sounds of "Dr. Bernard Harrison, please come to a white courtesy telephone for an important message."

I can still see him cackling his way through the concourse.

EPILOGUE

THE SUNRISE REFLECTING off the foothills of the Rockies was beautiful that early May morning. No dust, no swirling sand, no scorching heat. Just a friendly neighborhood dog sniffing for a place to soil my lawn.

I put my feet up on the same lawn chair as I had one morning a year, and a lifetime, ago. And once again I took in the sweet smell of the dew-covered grass that had been cut the night before. It was quiet, and the perfect time to talk with my dad.

I'd been back from Iraq for close to eight months and was slowly adjusting to life in the civilian world. I told him how good it felt to be home but still struggled as I tried to figure out how Iraq had changed me, or whether anything I'd done had changed Iraq. That it might be years before I came to any conclusions, if I ever did.

A few nights before, I had put in a long shift at work, ending my day with a crisis. A three-year-old boy's throat had swollen shut because of an allergic reaction. As his parents sprinted in with his blue, limp body, it seemed like the world had erupted in panic. Over the din of chaos, I heard a calm voice methodically ask for IVs, oxygen, Adrenalin, breathing tubes—the works. I was pleased to realize that the calm voice was mine. The kid did great; so did his doctor. No retching or vomit followed the case. After the child was awake and stable, I even went to my desk and ate a sandwich as I typed up the medical record.

Yet when my workday was done, I was sad. My drive home that evening was on dark, empty streets. How I longed to be with Rick kicking chunks of gravel across the compound as we made our way from the hospital tents to the barracks. Slinking in to see if any women were outside Bernard's door. Having Bill say, "Hey, dude, nice job there." Threatening Gerry's mustache with a razor. Calling Colonel Blok a "blockhead." Going back to my room to watch Mike lace up his sneakers for a late-night run. And Ian warning *me* not to snore.

God, I missed my friends. They had given me a richness few men ever experience. Our group has kept in touch—often at first, less as we ease back into civilian life. But even when we don't talk or e-mail, we are always secure in the knowledge that any of us would drop anything, at any time, if one of us needed help.

We have all had to deal with issues from the war. A few of us more than others, but each has carried home some bits of psychological debris from the carnage. The heaviest baggage included a mix of nightmares, moments of melancholy, short outbursts of temper, even a few tears when a particular song triggered a trip back to Iraq. Toughest of all was the feeling of being in a war one day, then abruptly deposited home the next and expected to simply pick up where we'd left off. It wasn't easy.

I told my dad how I still could only take small doses of TV and the newspapers. And when it came to talk radio, forget it. I was stunned at the name-calling, lack of civility, and just plain viciousness that often spewed from the dial. Worse yet was that it seemed many of the meanest talkers hadn't done a damn thing in their lives to serve our country.

I've never believed that you have to go to war to serve your country; that choice was mine and mine alone. But I had been raised to believe some form of service is important and that there are a lot of ways to do it, whether it's working at a soup kitchen, volunteering at a school, or just being a good neighbor. Service is what makes America the greatest country in the world. My dad showed me that when he gave up his Saturdays to put on magic shows for little kids living in the poorer sections of Newark or left early on Sundays to give an elderly widower a ride to church.

I thanked him for the lesson.

I also thanked him for teaching me the importance of honor, integrity, and humility, along with giving me advice about never being afraid to ask for help or extend a hand to offer help. I realized his words had, decades later, saved me in Iraq.

The diary of my war has been put away, tucked in a safe drawer alongside my dad's wallet. One day I'll pull them out and talk to my kids about what I did and what I saw, as well as what their grandfather went through. I just don't know when that time will be. But one thing we've already talked about is *why* I went.

It wasn't about penance or payback, those are nothing more than exhausting inventions of the human mind. I went because I was needed. And there is no greater honor than answering the call. A call, I realized, that isn't confined to war but is instead an ongoing, lifelong endeavor. My friends showed me that. So did my father, though I'm not sure he knew it at the time.

I stood up and took a final glance at the mountains, realizing it was time to finish our conversation. On this quiet spring morning, more than thirty years after his death, I told my dad that I finally understood. Even though he went through life burdened by guilt, he had, in his own way, taught me the lessons and given me the tools to conquer our perceived failures.

Real or imagined, our debts are now erased.

IAN NUNNALLY RETURNED to private practice as a general surgeon in Ohio. He is the director of his hospital's wound care program.

Robert Blok works as an anesthesiologist in North Carolina. He has volunteered to return to Iraq twice since our deployment in 2007.

Gerry Maloney works as an emergency physician in Cleveland. He got married shortly after his return to the States.

Mike Barron left his teaching position at Saint Louis University School of Medicine after our deployment and opened a family practice. He serves low-income families and those without health insurance.

Bill Stanton is an orthopedic surgeon in Fort Pierce, Florida. He was called back to duty in Iraq in June 2009.

Bernard Harrison is a cardiovascular and thoracic surgeon in Minneapolis. He is a pioneer in robotic surgery to treat heart disease.

Rick Reutlinger returned to Muskogee, Oklahoma, where he works as a general surgeon. He served a tour of duty in the spring of 2009 in Landstuhl, Germany, caring for soldiers wounded in Iraq and Afghanistan.

And I've returned to Littleton, Colorado, where I work as a family practitioner and an urgent care physician, and occasionally wield a surgical scalpel. I still never go anywhere without my cheat cards.

AUTHOR'S NOTE

ALTHOUGH MOST OF this book takes place in a combat zone, it's really not intended to be a tale of war. Instead, it is more of a story of life, thickly woven with the common threads of family and friendship. When you think about it, they are the most important things we possess, yet all too often go unappreciated until they are gone. For me, this experience put an exclamation point on the value of family and friends.

I relied heavily on notes, diaries, and e-mails to recount events. The manuscript was reviewed and discussed for accuracy and issues of confidentiality with colleagues and staff members of the 399th CSH. Dialogue, by necessity, was often written to the best of my recollection. Most importantly, the writing is a reflection of my perception of events in an often chaotic world. Any inaccuracies or errors are unintentional.

Descriptions of medical events and procedures were simplified for the lay reader. Military events were simplified so I could understand them. My apologies to the professionals in both fields.

We were given the honor and responsibility of caring for wounded human beings, most of whom we liked, some we did not, especially those who wanted to do us harm. In any case, it was important to preserve the dignity and privacy of anyone who came through our doors. To do so, it was often necessary to alter identifying characteristics and timelines. Yet there is no intent to mislead the reader. All of the stories, happy or sad, are true.

My special thanks to the family of David Heringes for allowing me to tell his heroic story.

With its musty tents and ramshackle buildings, our hospital wasn't much to look at on the outside. But the inside was filled with only the best.

The emergency room, or EMT as it was actually called, was expertly managed by Jack Twomey, Roger Boutin, and Bruce Courage. They never gave me grief over my shortcomings. The skillful team of registered nurses who always made the doctors look good included Rita Ed, Michelle Jacobs, Mark Thorbahn, and Steve Wetherill. The medics and flight nurses were Russell Albrycht, Ben Asay, Heather Belanger, Brian Brooks, John Clinton, Patrick Drake, James Elliott, Shannon Hansen, Chris Kretschmer, Katie Meloy, Lisa McCullough, Scott Moreau, Sharon Tetrault, Tim Verreault, Warren Ward, Hallie Whitmore, and Brian Yeager. You guys always made sure I knew who was really in charge (and it wasn't me).

Whether it be a bad trauma case, a tough surgery, or sick patient in post-op, we could always count on Robert Bento, Jeremy Bookman, Larry Brown, Jesse Burke, David Conti, Bob Czarniak, Brandon Gerry, Jossary Gerry, Allison Golden, Charles Pierce, Tim Rochfort, Brian Wallace, Stanley Warnock, and my favorite X-ray chief, Kirk Wolloff, among many others.

Always ready with lifesaving airways and oxygen were our nurse anesthetists, Mark Arturi, Leah Carpenter, Steve Lemoine, and Dean Losee. Thanks for the gas.

Physicians who were not official members of our group, but were invaluable in caring for patients or contributing to morning trivia were

Duane Luke, Kenny Smith, Andrew Torrance, and Gary Wheeler.

To the doctors who preceded our group at the 399th, a special salute. You set the standard for being the best.

And what can I say about the "Angels of Mercy" who staffed our ICU and wards? The patients, and we doctors, were blessed to have you.

In a war where you could wind up being assigned to a bad boss, we were lucky to have some good ones. Colonel Greg Quick held my hand without crushing it. Colonel Bryan Kelly kept the place from falling apart. LTC Rick Bailey was also one of the good guys.

Most importantly, we had leaders like Major General Ronald Silverman and Major General James Simmons, who in the midst of an unconventional war were able to see the big picture and ensure our soldiers got the best of care. And a special thanks to General David Petraeus, who didn't yell at me when I waved instead of saluting when we crossed paths in June 2007.

My 2004 deployment had its saviors as well. My commanders, Lieutenant Colonel Izzy Rommes and Brigadier General David Quantock, were models of honor, integrity, and wisdom, always leading from the front. Command Sergeant Major James Weaver could have chewed my inexperienced army butt to shreds, but instead took the time to patiently teach me how to act like an officer. I think the hair he pulled out has finally grown back.

My bodyguards, Bob Chenoweth and Steve Robinson, protected me on the road. Sergeant Rickey Hopson found me when I was lost. Captain Randy Conover kept me from getting lost again.

Although only crazy people jump out of perfectly functioning planes, I will be forever proud of being a soldier with the 160th MP Airborne Battalion and 16th MP Airborne Brigade.

Retired Colonel John Haynie was a one-man band tasked with keeping whining army doctors happy. His work at Fort Benning for deployed reservist physicians will earn him sainthood.

My friends on the home front deserve special mention, especially my coworkers at CBS4 in Denver, who never complained when I needed time off to be an army guy, or needed to juggle jobs with writing a book.

I never saw a "support the troops" decal on his truck, yet my neighbor Cam Tiffany put those words into action. He cut my lawn every week I was deployed. The little things mean a lot to a soldier away from home.

Gary Borgeson, Beth Henson, Kerry Mahoney, Huel Halliburton, and Ian Reutlinger were among the dozen civilians who reviewed the manuscript and steered the book back onto the road whenever I tried to drive it into a ditch.

Frank DeAngelis, you're more than a good principal, you are a good man.

Then there are the official book people. My editors at Simon & Schuster could have been a football coaches for all of the pats on the rump they gave to keep me in the game. Michele Bové was especially patient and kind with my repetitive questions and need for generous deadline extensions. Elisa Rivlin helped me navigate the legal land mines, especially those involving patient confidentiality and privacy. Finally, Larry Weissman, who truly is the world's best agent—as well as a stellar teacher of basic grammar.

My special thanks to all who serve or have served in times past. An even bigger hug goes to the families and loved ones who anxiously wait behind.

Finally, eternal thanks to the family who waited and fretted for me: Lucy, Moe, Piston, Yimster, and the Belle. You are the true blessings in my life.

ABOUT THE AUTHOR

Dr. Dave Hnida has been a practicing physician for more than twenty-five years. He also serves as the medical editor for KCNC-TV in Denver. He attended the University of Pennsylvania and spent his internship and residency at Rocky Mountain at Presbyterian/St. Luke's Medical Center. He currently lives in Colorado.